⚡ STEDMAN'S
Pocket Guide to
Medical Language

⚡ STEDMAN'S

Pocket Guide to
Medical Language

⬤ Wolters Kluwer | Lippincott Williams & Wilkins
    Health

Philadelphia · Baltimore · New York · London
Buenos Aires · Hong Kong · Sydney · Tokyo

Publisher: Julie K. Stegman
Senior Managing Editor: Heather Rybacki
Associate Managing Editor: Kristin Royer
Manufacturing Coordinator: Margie Orzech-Zeranko
Typesetter: Aptara, Inc.
Printer & Binder: C&C Offset Printing Company
Designer: Mike Zimmer

Printed in China

First Edition, 2009

Library of Congress Cataloging-in-Publication Data

Stedman's pocket guide to medical language. — 1st ed.
    p. ; cm.
ISBN 978-0-7817-9981-2
1. Medicine—Terminology—Handbooks, manuals, etc. I. Stedman,
Thomas Lathrop, 1853-1938. II. Title: Pocket guide to medical language.
    [DNLM: 1. Terminology as Topic. W 15 S8124 2009]
R123.S716 2009
610.1'4—dc22

2008022044

Table of Contents

Publisher's Preface

As the foundation for successful communication and understanding in any health care setting, medical terminology is the backbone of all medical disciplines. In a medical terminology course, students are typically taught word parts—prefixes, suffixes, and roots—which allow them to piece words together and understand their meaning. A key piece of medical terminology is the pronunciation of the words themselves since learning medical terminology, which is typically derived from Latin and Greek, is like learning a different language.

We received many requests to create a "pocket guide" for medical terminology. We have now published this guide to meet our customers' needs for a comprehensive, yet concise, portable format, enabling our readers to find the information they need quickly. It is our goal that *STEDMAN'S Pocket Guide to Medical Language* will provide students and professionals with a quick reference to key medical terminology and associated medical language information. Not meant to replace a core textbook, this quick reference will instead serve as a resource for the building blocks of medical terminology, offering guidance on how to form and pronounce medical terms, paired with a list of commonly encountered prefixes, suffixes, and combining forms. Dedicated sections feature commonly confused terminology (including a section on commonly confused drug names), abbreviations, acronyms, and symbols, and an overview of the medical record. Finally, *STEDMAN'S Pocket Guide* features valuable reference information such as: Healthcare Organization and Professional Designation Abbreviations, Spanish-English Medical Phrases, Laboratory Values, Diagnostic Tests and Procedures, Error-Prone Abbreviations, Complementary and Alternative Medicine

Terms, Internet Resources, the Top 200 Commonly Prescribed Drugs, and Drug Classifications and Therapeutic Uses.

Like any STEDMAN'S publication, a major focus of the development of this pocket guide, from the design to the format and style, was to present sought-after information in a format that would facilitate easy lookup and quick comprehension. To do this we have organized the information into easy to follow tables and lists. Sections are color-coded with running headers and footers to help orient you to the information on the page, and the book is small and portable enough to carry in your pocket.

As always, we at Lippincott Williams & Wilkins are grateful to all of our consultants from the medical, nursing, and health professions disciplines for their help in reviewing. Without them, none of the terminology presented here would be relevant or useful. We would first like to thank all of the customers who submitted this idea to us. Secondly, we would like to thank our review team who offered their input on the initial proposal and topics to be represented and the numerous reviewers who helped us select the title and topics. Finally, we are especially grateful to our editorial advisory board, who reviewed every page of this pocket guide to ensure the right information was presented accurately, comprehensively, and concisely.

We at Wolters Kluwer Health | Lippincott Williams & Wilkins strive to provide all of our readers—students, educators, and practitioners alike—with the most up-to-date and accurate medical language references. We welcome any suggestions you may have for improvements, changes, corrections, and additions—whatever makes it possible for this STEDMAN'S product to serve you better.

Julie K. Stegman	Heather Rybacki	Kristin Royer
Senior Publisher	Senior Managing Editor	Associate Managing Editor

Acknowledgments

Acknowledgments

Amy Semenchuk RN, BSN
Health Occupations
Department Chair
Rockford Business College
Rockford, IL

Lea M. Sims, CMT, AHDI-F
Director of Communications
& Publications
Association for Healthcare
Documentation Integrity
(AHDI)
Jacksonville, FL

Charlene Thiessen, MEd,
CMT, AHDI-F
Program Director, Medical
Transcription
Health Sciences Division
GateWay Community College
Phoenix, AZ

Carole A. Zeglin, MS, BS,
RMA
Director Medical Assistant
Program/Asst. Professor
Health Professions
Department
Westmoreland County
Community College
Youngwood, PA

Contributors

Robin Gardenhire, MA, ATC,
CSCS
Clinical Instructor
Georgia State University
Atlanta, GA

Diane Gilmore CMT, FAAMT
Director of Education
Transcription Relief Services
Institute
Springfield, Tennessee

Raymond Lukens
Editor and consultant,
Stedman's medical
dictionaries
Warren, MI

Manuscript Reviewers

Michelle Alarie

DeAnne Besetzny

Michelle Bing

Gerry Brasin

Rosalind Collazo

Grace Di Virgilio

Jean Fennema

Leora Fire

Margaret Fulsom

Cynthia Hart

Carolyn Helms

Lois R. Hine

Linda Karp

Donna Long

Noreen McCaustland

Cora Newcomb

Elizabeth Quick

Diane Sater

Navdeep Sekhon

Amy Semenchuk

Janet Sesser

Gina Stephens

Charlene Thiessen

Rod Tomczack

Explanatory Notes

Stedman's Pocket Guide to Medical Language provides students and professionals with an easy-to-use pocket resource for medical terminology and standard medical information. This book combines key components of learning medical terminology with a reference-based approach, using tables and reference lists to present information in an easy-to-find format. Please take a few minutes to review these Explanatory Notes, which will introduce you to the key sections of this book.

The **Medical Terminology** section serves as a resource for the building blocks of medical terminology. It provides guidance on how to form medical terms, introduces common prefixes, suffixes, and combining forms, and includes helpful pronunciation guidelines. This section also includes a comprehensive listing of complementary and alternative medical terms and their definitions and a glossary of useful Spanish expressions for the medical setting.

In **Abbreviations, Acronyms, & Symbols,** you will find tables with over a thousand commonly used medical abbreviations and symbols, plus hundreds of abbreviations for healthcare organizations and professional designations. It also includes the Joint Commission's list of dangerous abbreviations, acronyms, and symbols all in one convenient place.

The **Pharmacology** section identifies the top 200 prescription drugs and gives you quick access to a comprehensive classification of drugs and their therapeutic uses. Consult our look-alike and sound-alike section for hundreds of commonly confused drug names and refer to the error-prone pharmaceutical abbreviations for a listing of dose designations, abbreviations, and symbols that should be avoided to prevent harmful medication errors.

The **Lab and Diagnostic Information** puts common laboratory tests and the normal result values at your fingertips. This section also includes a thorough listing of diagnostic procedures and their indications.

In **Medical Records,** you have the opportunity to see how medical terms are used in clinical practice. This includes general guidelines for formatting a medical record, sample reports, and thorough explanations of the different types of medical reports, including clinic notes, history and physical reports, operative reports, consultation reports, discharge summaries, radiology reports, and pathology reports.

The **Internet Resources** classified by body region gives you easy access to a comprehensive list of web sites with up-to-date resources for further information.

Color **Body Plane** illustrations indicate major anatomic planes and radiographic positions, and the 16-page **Anatomy Atlas** features full-color illustrations of the major body systems, allowing you to identify and visualize the anatomy of body structures quickly and easily.

The **CD-ROM** included with the book includes interactive audio pronunciation drills that allow you to test your knowledge of word parts. With the Spanish-English pronunciation glossary, you can look up terms in Spanish or English and practice the Spanish pronunciations. Also included on the disc is an image bank, containing all the figures included in the book.

References

Cohen, BJ. *Medical Terminology: An Illustrated Guide, 5th Edition*. Baltimore: Lippincott Williams & Wilkins, 2007.

Nath, JL. *Using Medical Terminology: A Practical Approach*. Baltimore: Lippincott Williams & Wilkins, 2005.

Spanish English English-Spanish Medical Dictionary, 3rd Edition. Baltimore: Lippincott Williams & Wilkins, 2005.

Stedman's Alternative and Complementary Medicine Words, 2nd Edition. Baltimore: Lippincott Williams & Wilkins, 2005.

Stedman's Medical Abbreviations, Acronyms & Symbols, 4th Edition. Baltimore: Lippincott Williams & Wilkins, 2008.

Stedman's Medical Dictionary, 28th Edition. Baltimore: Lippincott Williams & Wilkins, 2006.

Stedman's Medical Dictionary for the Health Professions and Nursing, Illustrated, 6th Edition. Baltimore: Lippincott Williams & Wilkins, 2008.

Stedman's Medical Terminology Flash Cards. Baltimore: Lippincott Williams & Wilkins, 2005.

Willis MC. *Medical Terminology A Programmed Learning Approach to the Language of Health Care, 2nd Edition*. Baltimore: Lippincott Williams & Wilkins, 2007.

Abbreviations, Acronyms, & Symbols

The Official "Do Not Use" List. The Joint Commission. Available at: http://www.jointcommission.org/NR/rdonlyres/2329F8F5-6EC5-4E21-B932-54B2B7D53F00/0/dnu_list.pdf. Accessed June 10, 2008.

Lab and Diagnostic Information

Burtis CA, Ashwood ER. eds. *Tietz Textbook of Clinical Chemistry, 3rd Edition*. Philadelphia: WB Saunders, 1998.

Children's Hospital, St. Louis, The Department of Clinical Laboratories, High Density Lipoprotein Lipid Panel: Cholesterol, HDL, Cholesterol, LDL (calculated), Cholesterol, Total, Triglycerides, Parathyroid Hormone (PTH). Available at http://webserver01.bjc.org/slch/pro/Professional.htm?http://webserver01.bjc.org/labtestguide/Lab%20Test%20Guidebook/slchlabsiteoutline.htm. Accessed April 20, 2004.

Clinical chemistry laboratory: Reference range values in clinical chemistry. Professional services manual. Baltimore, Department of Pathology, University of Maryland Medical System, 1999.

Harmening DM, ed. *Hematologic Values in Chemical Hematology and Fundamentals of Hemostasis, 2nd Edition*. Philadelphia: FA Davis, 1992.

Laboratory Corporation of America, Erythrocyte Sedimentation Rate, Westergren. Available at http://www.labcorp.com/datasets/labcorp/html/chapter/mono/he005000.htm. Accessed April 20, 2004.

Laboratory Corporation of America. Fecal Fat. Quantitative. Available at http://www.labcorp.com/datasets/labcorp/html/chapter/mono/sc008000.htm. Accessed April 20, 2004.

National cholesterol education program: Report of the expert panel on detection, evaluation, and treatment of high blood cholesterol in adults. Arch Intern Med 1988;148:36-69.

Triglyceride, high density lipoprotein and coronary heart disease. National Institute of Health Consensus Statement, NIH Consensus Development Conference, 1992;10(2).

University of Texas Health Center at San Antonio. Neonatal Bilirubin. Available at http://labs-sec.uhs-sa.com/clinical_ext/dols/soprefrange.aps. Accessed April 20, 2004.

University of Texas Medical Branch. Erythrocyte Sedimentation Rate, Wintrobe. Available at http://www.utmb.edu/lsg/LabSurvivalGuide/hem/Sedimentation_Rate.htm. Accessed April 20, 2004.

University of Virginia Children's Medical Center. Therapy Review: Warfarin (Coumadin®). Pediatric Pharmacotherapy. January 1995;1(5):386. Available at http://www.people.virginia.edu/~smb4v/cmchome.html. Accessed April 20, 2004.

Warfarin Therapy in Children Who Require Long-Term Total Parenteral Nutrition. Pediatrics [electronic article]. November 2003;112(5):386. Available at http://pediatrics.aappublications.org/cgi/content/full/112/5/e386. Accessed April 20, 2004.

Pharmacology

Error-Prone Abbreviation List. Institute for Safe Medication Practices. Available at: http://www.ismp.org/Tools/errorprone-abbreviations.pdf. Accessed June 10, 2008.

Springhouse Nurse's Drug Guide, 2006. Philadelphia: Lippincott Williams & Wilkins, 2006.

Top 200 Prescription Drugs of 2007. *Pharmacy Times*. May 2008; 20-24. Available at: http://www.pharmacytimes.com/issues/articles/2008-05_003.asp. Accessed June 10, 2008.

Image Sources

From *Stedman's Medical Dictionary, 28th Edition*. Baltimore: Lippincott Williams & Wilkins 2006. (Radiographic projections)

From *Stedman's Medical Dictionary for the Health Professions and Nursing, Illustrated, 6th Edition*. Baltimore: Lippincott Williams & Wilkins 2008. (Anatomical position and directional references, Positions on the operating table)

From Willis MC. *Medical Terminology: A Programmed Learning Approach to the Language of Health Care, 2nd Edition*. Baltimore: Lippincott Williams & Wilkins, 2007. (Anatomical position with body planes)

All artwork in the anatomy insert, *Anatomical Chart Company*. All rights reserved.

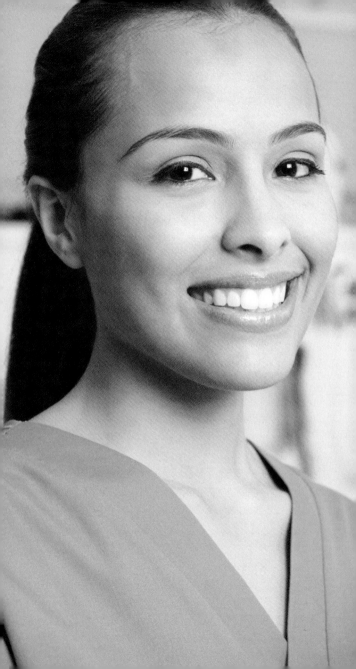

Medical Terminology

Word Building

Most medical terms have three basic component parts.

^P ^R ^S

endoabdominal

1. The **root** is the foundation or subject of each medical word. It establishes the basic meaning of the word and is the part to which modifying prefixes and suffixes are added.

2. A **suffix** is a short word part or series of parts added at the end of a root that modifies and gives essential meaning to the root.

3. A **prefix** is a short word part added before a root to modify its meaning. A prefix is not always present.

In addition, some medical terms are constructed using a combining vowel. A **combining vowel** is used when a medical term has more than one root or to join root to suffix. The most common combining vowel is the letter "o." When the combining vowel is written with the root, it is called a **combining form**.

There are five basic rules for constructing terms:

$$\overset{\text{R}}{\text{micr}} \overset{}{\text{o}} \overset{\text{S}}{\text{scope}}$$

1. A combining vowel is used to join root to root, as well as root to any suffix beginning with a consonant. For example, in the term microscope, **micr** is a root and **scope** is a suffix. Add "o," the combining vowel, to join root to suffix.

$$\overset{\text{R}}{\text{ceph}} \overset{\text{S}}{\text{algia}}$$

2. A combining vowel is not used before a suffix that begins with a vowel. For example, in the term cephalgia, **ceph** is the root and **algia** is the suffix, which begins with a vowel. No combining vowel is used.

$$\overset{\text{R}}{\text{card}} \overset{\text{S}}{\text{itis}}$$

3. If the root ends in a vowel and the suffix begins with the same vowel, drop the final vowel from the root and do not use a combining vowel. For example, in the term carditis, the root **cardi** ends in "i" and the suffix **itis** begins with "i." The "i" in **cardi** is therefore removed and the root and suffix are joined with no combining vowel.

$$\overset{\text{R}}{\text{gastr}} \overset{}{\text{o}} \overset{\text{R}}{\text{esophag}} \overset{\text{S}}{\text{eal}}$$

4. Most often, a combining vowel is inserted between two roots, even when the second root begins with a vowel. For example, in the term gastroesophageal, both **gastr** and **esophag** are roots. They are joined with the combining vowel "o," even though **esophag** begins with a vowel.

^P   ^R
par|esthesia

5. Occasionally, when a prefix ends in a vowel and the root begins with a vowel, the final vowel is dropped from the prefix. For example, in the term paresthesia, **para** is the prefix ending in a vowel and **esthesia** is the root. The final "a" in the prefix is dropped when forming this word.

All of these rules have exceptions. A medical dictionary is the best place to check for the correct spelling, formation, or precise meaning of a term. Some exceptions to note are:

^R   ^R
ovi|duct

1. Terms can be formed by a root alone or by a combination of roots. For example, in the term oviduct, both **ovi** and **duct** are roots, which combine together to form a medical term.

^P   ^S
meta|stasis

2. Terms can be formed by the combination of a prefix and suffix alone. For example, in the term metastasis, **meta** is a prefix and **stasis** is a suffix.

Spelling Medical Terms

When using medical terms, one must pay very close attention to how a term is used and how it is spelled. Even a difference of one letter in a word can change a term's meaning. For example, the root **cyt** means "cells," whereas **cyst** means "bladder." In addition, **thym** is the root for the thymus gland, whereas **thyr** is the root for the thyroid gland.

Keep in mind the following points when spelling medical terms.

1. Some words sound the same but are spelled differently and have different meanings. Determine how the word is used in context to know how to spell the term. For example:

ileac	**iliac**
(relating to the ileus)	(relating to the ilium)
humerus	**humorous**
(a bone of the arm)	(funny)

2. Other words sound similar but are spelled differently and have different meanings. For example:

abasia	**astasia**
(inability to walk)	(inability to stand)
brachial	**bronchial**
(relating to the arm)	(relating to the bronchi)
decimate	**desiccate**
(to kill or destroy)	(to dry thoroughly)

3. When letters are silent in a term, they risk being omitted when spelling the word. For example:

   • The letter combination **pt** has a **t** sound if found at the beginning of a term (e.g., ptyalography)

   • The letter combination **ph** has an **f** sound (e.g., aphagia)

   • The letter combination **ps** has an **s** sound (e.g., psychosis)

4. When you add a suffix to a word ending in **x**, the **x** is changed to a **g** or a **c**.

   • If there is a consonant before the **x** (e.g., the letter combination **nx** or **yx**), the **x** is changed to a **g**. For example, phalanx becomes phalangeal and coccyx becomes coccygeal.

   • If a vowel comes before the **x** (e.g., the letter combination **ex** or **ix**), the **x** is changed to a **c**. For example, vertex becomes vertices and appendix becomes appendicitis.

5. When you add a suffix beginning with **rh** to a root, the **r** is doubled.

   • The root **lapar/o** and the suffix **-rhaphy** become laparorrhaphy.

   • The root **men/o** and the suffix **-rhagia** become menorrhagia.

6. Some words have more than one accepted spelling. For example:

   • orthopedic/orthopaedic

   • leukocyte/leucocyte

Word Etymology

Etymology is the study of the origin of words. Like many medical terms, it has Greek origins: **étymos** (or, the actual meaning of a word) and **lògos** (meaning science). Thus, it is the science of the construction of words from other words and parts of other words.

Most medical terms are put together from roots that derive from Latin and Greek, although much changed over the centuries. These roots are used in conjunction with combining forms, like suffixes and prefixes, to produce words that will convey the meaning for the many thousands of scientific and medically specific nomenclatures needed to describe body parts, diseases, and procedures.

As medical knowledge grows, so does the vocabulary used to describe it. New words are created using the component forms mentioned above. Thus, etymology, which is normally found at the end of a definition in a dictionary, may be the most useful part of learning a new word. The same root will carry the same meaning, even if used in different combinations. Therefore, if you learn the etymology of the word forms **myo** (related to muscle) and **cardio** (related to the heart), the meaning of the word myocardium (the middle layer of the heart, the cardiac muscle) is self-explanatory.

Rules of Pronunciation

Practice is the main key for learning how to properly pronounce a medical term. The information below will guide you through the sounds some letters or letter combinations take on. For more information and audio pronunciations, please refer to the CD that accompanies this book.

Letter	Sounds like	Examples
c (before a, o, u)	k	calorie, carotid
c (before e, i)	s	cecum, cirrhosis
ch	k	chloroform, chord
dys	dis	dyslexia
eu	u	eupnea
g (before a, o, u)	g	gate, gastric
g (before e, i)	j	gel
gn	n	gnat
ph	f	phlebitis, phobia
pn	n	pneumonia
ps		psychosis
pt	t	ptosis, pterygium
rh, rrh	r	rhyme, menorrhagia
x (as the first letter in a word)	z	Xerox

Forming Plurals

Plurals are usually formed by adding "s" or "es" to the end of a singular form.

Exceptions are:

Singular ending	Example	Plural ending	Example
-a	bulla	-ae	bullae
-is	crisis	-es	crises
-ma	stoma	-mata	stomata
-on	ganglion	-a	ganglia
-um	speculum	-a	specula
-us*	radius	-i	radii
-ax	pneumothorax	-aces	pneumothoraces
-ex	cortex	-ices	cortices
-y	autopsy	-ies	autopsies

*The words virus and sinus follow the general rules of making plurals (viruses and sinuses); they are not exceptions.

Prefixes, Suffixes, and Combining Forms

The following is a list of commonly used medical term prefixes, suffixes, and roots. Prefixes are followed by a hyphen, suffixes are preceded by a hyphen, and roots are separated from their combining vowel with a slash.

Word Part	Meaning
a-	not, without, lack of, absence
ab-	away from
abdomin/o	abdomen
-ac	pertaining to
acous, acus	sound, hearing
acr/o	extremity, end
ad-	toward, near
aden/o	gland
adip/o	fat
adren/o	adrenal gland, epinephrine
adrenal/o	adrenal gland
adrenocortic/o	adrenal cortex
aer/o	air, gas
-al	pertaining to
alg/o, algi/o, algesi/o	pain
-algia, -algesia	pain
ambly/o	dim
amni/o	amnion
amyl/o	starch
an-	not, without, lack of, absence
an/o	anus
andr/o	male

Word Part	Meaning
angi/o	vessel
ante-	before
anti-	against
aort/o	aorta
-ar	pertaining to
arter/o, arteri/o	artery
arteriol/o	arteriole
arthr/o	joint
-ary	pertaining to
-ase	enzyme
atlant/o	atlas
atri/o	atrium
audi/o	hearing
auto-	self
azo-, azot/o	nitrogenous compounds
bacill/i, bacill/o	bacillus
bacteri/o	bacterium
balan/o	glans penis
bar/o	pressure
bi-	two, twice
bil/i	bile
-blast, blast/o	immature cell, productive cell, embryonic cell
blephar/o	eyelid
brachi/o	arm
brachy-	short
brady-	slow
bronch/i, bronch/o	bronchus
bronchiol/o	bronchiole
bucc/o	cheek
burs/o	bursa
calc/i	calcium
cali/o, calic/o	calyx

2

2

Word Part	Meaning
-capnia	carbon dioxide (level of)
carcin/o	cancer, carcinoma
cardi/o	heart
cec/o	cecum
-cele	hernia, localized dilation
celi/o	abdomen
-centesis	puncture, tap
cephal/o	head
cerebell/o	cerebellum
cerebr/o	cerebrum
cervic/o	neck, cervix
cheil/o	lip
chem/o	chemical
chol/e, chol/o	bile, gall
cholangi/o	bile duct
cholecyst/o	gallbladder
choledoch/o	common bile duct
chondr/o	cartilage
chori/o, choroid/o	choroid
chrom/o, chromat/o	color, stain
chron/o	time
circum-	around
-clasis, -clasia	breaking
clitor/o, clitorid/o	clitoris
coccyg/o	coccyx
cochle/o	cochlea (of inner ear)
col/o, colon/o	colon
colp/o	vagina
contra-	against, opposed
copro-	feces
corne/o	cornea
cortic/o	outer portion, cerebral cortex

Word Part	Meaning
cost/o	rib
counter-	opposite, against
crani/o	skull, cranium
cry/o	cold
crypt/o	hidden
cyan-, cyano-	blue
cycl/o	ciliary body, ciliary muscle (of eye)
cyst/o, cyst/i	filled sac or pouch, cyst, bladder, urinary bladder
cyt/o, -cyte	cell
dacry/o	tear, lacrimal apparatus
dacryocyst/o	lacrimal sac
dactyl/o	finger, toe
de-	down, without, removal, loss
dent/o, dent/i	tooth, teeth
derm/o, dermat/o	skin
-desis	binding, fusion
dextr/o	right
di-	two, twice
dia-	through
-dilation, -dilatation	expansion, widening
dipl/o	double
dis-	absence, removal, separation
duoden/o	duodenum
dys-	abnormal, painful, difficult
ec-	out, outside
-ectasia, -ectasis	dilation, dilatation, distention
ecto-	out, outside
-ectomy	excision, surgical removal

Word Part	Meaning
-edema	accumulation of fluid, swelling
electr/o	electricity
embry/o	embryo
-emesis	vomiting
-emia	condition of blood
encephal/o	brain
endo-	in, within
endocrin/o	endocrine
enter/o	intestine
epi-	on, over
epididym/o	epididymis
episi/o	vulva
equi-	equal, same
erg/o	work
erythr/o	red, red blood cell
erythrocyt/o	red blood cell
esophag/o	esophagus
-esthesia, esthesi/o	sensation
eu-	true, good, easy, normal
exo-	away from, outside
extra-	outside
fasci/o	fascia
ferri-, ferr/o	iron
fet/o	fetus
fibr/o	fiber
-form	like, resembling
galact/o	milk
gangli/o, ganglion/o	ganglion
gastr/o	stomach
-gen, -genesis	origin, formation

Word Part	Meaning
ger/e, ger/o	old age
-geusia	sense of taste
gingiv/o	gum, gingiva
gli/o	neuroglia
glomerul/o	glomerulus
gloss/o	tongue
gluc/o	glucose
glyc/o	sugar, glucose
gnath/o	jaw
goni/o	angle
-gram	record of data
-graph	instrument for recording data
-graphy	act of recording data
-gravida	pregnant woman
gyn/o, gynec/o	woman
hem/o, hemat/o	blood
hemi-	half, one side
-hemia	condition of blood
hepat/o	liver
hetero-	other, different, unequal
hidr/o	sweat, perspiration
hist/o, histi/o	tissue
homo-, homeo-	same, unchanging
hydr/o	water, fluid
hyper-	over, excess, increased, abnormally high
hypn/o	sleep
hypo-	under, below, decreased, abnormally low
hyster/o	uterus
-ia, -iasis	condition of
-ian	specialist

Word Part	Meaning
iatr/o	physician
-iatrics, -iatry	medical specialty
-ic, -ical	pertaining to
-ics	medical specialty
-ile	pertaining to
ile/o, ili/o	ileum
im-	not
immun/o	immunity, immune system
in-	not
in/o	fiber, muscle fiber
infra-	below
insul/o	pancreatic islets
inter-	between
irit/o, irid/o	iris
-ism	condition of
iso-	equal, same
-ist	specialist
-itis	inflammation
jejun/o	jejunum
juxta-	near, beside
kal/i	potassium
kary/o	nucleus
kerat/o	cornea, keratin, horny layer of skin
kin/o, kinesi/o, kinet/o	movement
labi/o	lip
labyrinth/o	labyrinth (inner ear)
lacrim/o	tear, lacrimal apparatus
lact/o	milk
-lalia	speech, babble
lapar/o	abdominal wall

Word Part	Meaning
laryng/o	larynx
lent/i	lens
-lepsy	seizure
leuk/o	white, colorless, white blood cell
leukocyt/o	white blood cell
-lexia	reading
lingu/o	tongue
lip/o	fat, lipid
-listhesis	slipping
lith/o	calculus, stone
-logy	study of
lumb/o	lumbar region, lower back
lymph/o	lymph, lymphatic system, lymphocyte
lymphaden/o	lymph node
lymphangi/o	lymphatic vessel
lymphocyt/o	lymphocyte
-lysis	separation, loosening, dissolving, destruction
-lytic	dissolving, reducing, loosening
macro-	large, abnormally large
mal-	bad, poor
-malacia	softening
mamm/o	breast, mammary gland
-mania	excited state, obsession
mast/o	breast, mammary gland
medull/o	inner part, medulla oblongata, spinal cord
mega-, megalo-	large, abnormally large

Word Part	Meaning
-megaly	enlargement
melan/o	dark, black, melanin
men/o	month, menstruation
mening/o, meninge/o	meninges
meso-	middle
-meter	instrument for measuring
metr/o, metr/i	uterus
-metry	measurement of
micro-	small, one millionth
-mimetic	mimicking, simulating
mono-	one
morph/o	form, structure
muc/o	mucus, mucous membrane
multi-	many
muscul/o	muscle
my/o	muscle
myc/o	fungus, mold
myel/o	bone marrow, spinal cord
myring/o	tympanic membrane
myx/o	mucus
narc/o	stupor, unconsciousness
nas/o	nose
nat/i	birth
natr/i	sodium
-necrosis	death of tissue
neo-	new
nephr/o	kidney
neur/o, neur/i	nervous system, nerve
noct/i	night
non-	not
normo-	normal
nucle/o	nucleus

Word Part	Meaning
nyct/o	night, darkness
ocul/o	eye
odont/o	tooth, teeth
-odynia	pain
-oid	like, resembling
olig/o	few, scanty, deficiency of
-oma	tumor
onc/o	tumor
onych/o	nail
oo-	ovum
oophor/o	ovary
ophthalm/o	eye
-opia	eye, vision
-opsia	vision
opt/o	eye, vision
or/o	mouth
orchid/o, orchi/o	testis
orth/o	straight, correct, upright
-ory	pertaining to
osche/o	scrotum
-ose	sugar
-osis	condition of
-osmia	sense of smell
oste/o	bone
ot/o	ear
-ous	pertaining to
ov/o, ovul/o	ovum
ovari/o	ovary
ox/y	oxygen, sharp, acute
-oxia	oxygen (level of)
pachy-	thick
palat/o	palate

Word Part	Meaning
palpebr/o	eyelid
pan-	all
pancreat/o	pancreas
papill/o	nipple
para-	near, beside, abnormal
parathyr/o, parathyroid/o	parathyroid
-paresis	partial paralysis
path/o, -pathy	disease, any disease of
ped/o	foot, child
pelvi/o	pelvis
-penia	decrease in, deficiency of
per-	through
peri-	around
perine/o	perineum
peritone/o	peritoneum
-pexy	surgical fixation
phac/o, phak/o	lens
phag/o	eat, ingest
pharmac/o	drug, medicine
pharyng/o	pharynx
-phasia	speech
-phil, -philic	attracting, absorbing
phleb/o	vein
-phobia	fear
phon/o	sound, voice
-phonia	voice
phot/o	light
phren/o	diaphragm
phrenic/o	phrenic nerve
phyt/o	plant

Word Part	Meaning
-plasia	formation, molding, development
-plasty	plastic repair, plastic surgery, reconstruction
-plegia	paralysis
pleur/o	pleura
-pnea	breathing
pneum/o, pneumat/o	air, gas, lung, respiration
pneumon/o	lung
pod/o	foot
-poiesis	formation, production
poikilo-	varied, irregular
poly-	many, much
post-	after, behind
pre-	before, in front of
presby/o	old
primi-	first
pro-	before, in front of
proct/o	rectum
prostat/o	prostate
prote/o	protein
pseudo-	false
psych/o	mind
-ptosis	dropping, downward displacement, prolapse
ptysis	spitting
pulm/o, pulmon/o	lung
pupill/o	pupil
py/o	pus
pyel/o	renal pelvis
pylor/o	pylorus

Word Part	Meaning
pyr/o, pyret/o	fever, fire
quadri-	four
rachi/o	spine
radi/o	radiation, x-ray
radicul/o	root of spinal nerve
re-	again, back
rect/o	rectum
ren/o	kidney
reticul/o	network
retin/o	retina
retro-	behind, backward
rhabd/o	rod, muscle cell
-rhage, -rhagia	bursting forth, profuse flow, hemorrhage
-rhaphy	surgical repair, suture
-rhexis	rupture
rhin/o	nose
-rrhea	flow, discharge
sacchar/o	sugar
sacr/o	sacrum
salping/o	tube, oviduct, eustachian (auditory) tube
-schisis	fissure, splitting
scler/o	hard, sclera (of eye)
-sclerosis	hardening
-scope	instrument for viewing or examining
-scopy	examination of
seb/o	sebum, sebaceous gland
semi-	half, partial
sept/o	septum, partition, dividing wall

Word Part	Meaning
sial/o	saliva, salivary gland, salivary duct
sider/o	iron
sigmoid/o	sigmoid colon
sinistr/o	left
-sis	condition of
somat/o	body
-some	body, small body
somn/i, somn/o	sleep
son/o	sound, ultrasound
-spasm	sudden contraction, cramp
sperm/i, spermat/o	semen, spermatozoa
-spermia	condition of semen
spir/o	breathing
splen/o	spleen
spondyl/o	vertebra
staped/o, stapedi/o	stapes
staphyl/o	grapelike cluster, staphylococcus
-stasis	suppression, stoppage
steat/o	fatty
-stenosis	narrowing, constriction
steth/o	chest
sthen/o	strength
stomat/o	mouth
-stomy	surgical creation of an opening
strepto-	twisted chain, streptococcus
sub-	below, under
super-	above, excess
supra-	above

Word Part	Meaning
syn-, sym-	together
synov/i	synovial joint, synovial membrane
tachy-	rapid
tax/o	order, arrangement
tel/e, tel/o	end
ten/o, tendin/o	tendon
terat/o	malformed fetus
test/o	testis, testicle
tetra-	four
thalam/o	thalamus
therm/o	heat, temperature
thorac/o	chest, thorax
thromb/o	blood clot
thrombocyt/o	platelet, thrombocyte
thym/o	thymus gland
thyr/o, thyroid/o	thyroid
toc/o	labor
-tome	instrument for incising (cutting)
-tomy	incision, cutting
ton/o	tone
tonsill/o	tonsil
tox/o, toxic/o	poison, toxin
-toxin	poison
trache/o	trachea
trans-	through
tri-	three
trich/o	hair
-tripsy	crushing
troph/o, -trophy, -trophia	feeding, growth, nourishment
-tropic	turning toward, having an affinity for

Word Part	Meaning
tympan/o	tympanic cavity (middle ear), tympanic membrane
un-	not
uni-	one
ur/o	urine, urinary tract
-uresis	urination
ureter/o	ureter
urethr/o	urethra
-uria	condition of urine, urination
urin/o	urine
uter/o	uterus
uve/o	uvea (of eye)
uvul/o	uvula
vagin/o	sheath, vagina
valv/o, valvul/o	valve
varic/o	twisted and swollen vein, varix
vas/o	vessel, duct, vas deferens
vascul/o	vessel
ven/o, ven/i	vein
ventricul/o	cavity, ventricle
vertebr/o	vertebra, spinal column
vesic/o	urinary bladder
vesicul/o	seminal vesicle
vestibul/o	vestibule, vestibular apparatus (of ear)
vir/o	virus
vulv/o	vulva
xanth/o	yellow
xen/o	foreign, strange
xer/o	dry
-y	condition of

Complementary and Alternative Medicine Terms

acupressure A treatment involving the application of pressure to those areas of the body used in acupuncture.

acupuncture A traditional Chinese therapeutic technique involving puncturing the skin with fine needles to influence the flow of *qi* (vital energy).

African medicine Traditional African therapeutic techniques, based on naturopathic medicine, designed to treat the physical, mental, and spiritual causes of disease.

Alexander technique A system of educational therapy involving the use of minimal effort for maximum movement to improve posture and alleviate pain.

allopathy A term used to describe conventional Western medicine, in contrast to alternative or complementary medicine.

Alpha Calm Therapy A therapeutic technique involving guided imagery and hypnosis.

alternative medicine A general term for therapeutic practices that fall outside the realm of evidence-based mainstream medicine and are intended as replacements for conventional medical treatments. Alternative medical therapies fall into five main groups: complete medical systems (e.g., homeopathy and Chinese medicine), mind-body interventions (e.g., visualization and yoga), manipulative and body-based methods (e.g., chiropractic and massage), biologically based therapies (e.g., herbalism and macrobiotics), and energy therapies (e.g., qi gong and vibrational medicine).

Ama Deus A South American Indian system of healing.

apitherapy Treatment of illness involving the administration of honeybee stings.

applied kinesiology The use of muscle testing to identify illness. Applied kinesiology is based on the theory that weakness in certain muscles is associated with imbalances in the body.

aromatherapy A form of treatment involving the use of concentrated oils from plants with healing properties.

art therapy A therapy involving the use of artistic expression to promote emotional well-being.

Ayurveda A form of natural medicine, traditional in India, which provides an integrated approach to preventing and treating illness through lifestyle intervention and natural therapy. It involves *nadis* (canals) that carry *prana* (energy) throughout the body, *chakras* (centers of consciousness) that connect body and soul, and *marmas* (points on the body beneath which vital structures connect).

Bach flower therapy A system of diagnosis and treatment developed by British physician Edward Bach, which involves the use of flower essences.

biofeedback A method of treatment that uses monitors to help patients recognize physiological information of which they are normally unaware. Using this method, patients can learn to consciously control involuntary bodily processes such as blood pressure, temperature, gastrointestinal functioning, and brain wave activity.

bodywork A group of therapeutic techniques that involve exercising or manipulating the body to produce healing.

Bowen technique A form of bodywork developed by Australian Tom Bowen, in which certain body areas are lightly touched to stimulate energy flow.

chelation therapy The administration of chelating agents (drugs that bind to and remove certain materials from the body) to treat or prevent illness.

Chinese medicine An ancient health care system, traditional in China, based on the concept that disease results from disruption of *qi* (vital energy) and imbalance of *yin* (negative energy) and *yang* (positive energy). Chinese medicine encompasses several therapies, including herbal and nutritional therapy, restorative physical exercises, meditation, acupuncture, and massage.

chiropractic A diagnostic and therapeutic system based on the concept that disease results from nervous system malfunction. Treatment involves manipulation and adjustment of body structures, particularly the spinal column, to relieve local and distant physical ailments.

complementary medicine A general term for therapeutic techniques that are intended to accompany and support mainstream evidence-based medical treatments.

craniosacral therapy A diagnostic and therapeutic system in which the bones of the skull are manipulated to remove impediments to cerebrospinal fluid flow, with the goals of stress relief, pain alleviation, and overall health improvement.

cupping A treatment that consists of attaching a cup to the skin and evacuating the air within to increase local blood flow.

curanderismo A Mexican-American traditional form of medicine encompassing acupuncture and homeopathy (from the Spanish *curar*, meaning to treat or cure).

Feldenkrais method A form of bodywork developed by Israeli physicist Moshe Feldenkrais, which includes private instruction (functional integration) and group instruction (awareness through movement).

Gerson therapy A dietary therapy developed by German physician Max Gerson, which involves sodium restriction, potassium supplementation, fat restriction, periodic protein restriction, and coffee enemas.

guided imagery A technique in which patients imagine or visualize certain scenarios to improve health or promote healing.

herbal medicine The practice of creating or prescribing plant-derived remedies for medical conditions.

holistic medicine A general term for therapies, such as yoga, that emphasize the unity of body, mind, and spirit.

homeopathy A therapeutic system based on the concept that a disease may be treated with minute doses of drugs that cause the same symptoms in healthy people as the disease itself.

Substances are potentized (diluted) to prepare remedies (pharmacologic therapies) for patients. Homeopathic medicine is practiced in a holistic fashion, incorporating the elements of body, mind, and spirit.

hydrotherapy The internal and external use of water for the treatment of disease.

hypnosis The induction of trance states to treat a wide variety of conditions such as substance addiction, pain, and phobias.

Kneipping A system of natural healing developed by Dominican priest Sebastian Kneipp, based on the principles of hydrotherapy and herbalism.

Korean medicine A form of medicine traditional in Korea, which encompasses acupuncture and moxibustion.

macrobiotics A vegetarian dietary therapy promoting health and longevity.

magnet therapy A therapy in which magnetic fields are applied to the body using magnetic field-generating machines, magnetic mattresses, or blankets.

massage therapy A therapeutic system involving muscle manipulation to reduce tension and pain, promote relaxation, or diminish symptoms of muscular or neurologic diseases.

meridian therapy A therapeutic method that involves rhythmic breathing, visualization, and moving one's hands along meridians, which are lines along the body said to represent channels through which *qi* (vital energy) flows.

moxibustion A traditional Chinese medical therapy that involves burning *moxa* (mugwort or *Artemisia vulgaris*) and placing it at certain points on the body to stimulate *qi* (vital energy).

naturopathy A therapeutic system involving the use of heat, water, light, air, and massage for treatment of disease. The discipline is comprised of a number of alternative medical therapies, including homeopathy, herbal medicine, acupuncture, hydrotherapy, and manipulative therapy.

orthomolecular medicine A therapeutic modality and preventative medicine strategy involving the use of natural substances found in food (such as vitamins, amino acids, and minerals) to treat and prevent disease. Supplementation with relatively large doses of vitamins (megavitamin therapy) is sometimes used.

qigong A component of Chinese medicine that uses physical movement, breathing regulation, and meditation to achieve optimum health. From the Mandarin *qi* (breath) and *gong* (work or technique).

reflexology The practice of stimulating certain points on the body, most commonly on the feet, to improve health.

Reiki A therapy based on the theory that as spiritual energy is channeled through a Reiki practitioner, the patient's body and spirit are healed. From the Japanese *rein* (spirit or soul) and *kid* (energy or life force).

Rolfing A form of myofascial massage developed by American chemist Ida P. Rolf, which involves deep soft-tissue manipulation to release stored tension and manually realign body structures.

shiatsu A massage technique that originated in Japan, in which the thumbs, palms, fingers, and elbows are used to place pressure at certain points on the body.

tai chi An ancient Chinese martial art involving a combination of intentional leveraged movement and focused breathing to improve health and longevity.

Trager A form of bodywork developed by Dr. Milton Trager, which combines physical movement with meditation.

vibrational medicine A general term for therapeutic modalities based on the concept that disease originates in subtle energy systems, which are affected by environmental, nutritional, spiritual, and emotional factors. Examples of vibrational medicine therapies include acupuncture, aromatherapy, homeopathy, crystal healing, and orthomolecular medicine.

yoga A system of exercises for the improvement of physical and spiritual health, derived from Hindu tradition.

Commonly Confused Medical Terms

Term	Meaning
abasia	inability to walk
astasia	inability to stand
abneural	away from the neural axis
abnormal	strange, not normal
adapts	adjusts to a situation or circumstance
adeps	denoting fat or adipose tissue
aggressin	a substance of microbial origin postulated to inhibit the resistance mechanisms of the host
aggression	a domineering, forceful, or verbal assault or physical action toward another person
anabiotic	1) restorative; 2) a powerful stimulant
antibiotic	1) relating to antibiosis; 2) prejudicial to life; 3) a soluble substance derived from a mold or bacterium that inhibits the growth of other microorganisms
anaclitic	leaning or depending upon
analytic	relating to analysis
anecdote	report of clinical experience based on individual cases rather than organized investigation
antidote	an agent that neutralizes or counteracts the effects of poison
anergy	1) inability to generate sensitivity reaction to substances expected to be antigenic; 2) lack of energy
energy	vim and vigor

Term	Meaning
anorexia	an eating disorder
anorexiant	appetite suppressant
anoxia	without oxygen
anuresis	inability to urinate
enuresis	involuntary discharge or leakage of urine
aphagia	inability to eat
aphasia	impaired or absent production of speech, writing, or signs due to an acquired lesion of the dominant cerebral hemisphere
aplasia	defective development or congenital absence of an organ or tissue
apraxia	a disorder of voluntary movement consisting of impairment in the performance of skilled or purposeful movements
ataxia	inability to coordinate muscle activity during voluntary movement
asthenia	weakness or debility
sthenia	a condition of activity and apparent force
asoma	a fetus with only one rudimentary body
asthma	an inflammatory disease of the lungs
auxiliary	functioning in an augmenting capacity
axillary	relating to the axilla
axion	the brain and spinal cord
axon	the single process of a nerve cell

Term	Meaning
bacterid	persistent eruption of discrete pustules of the palms and soles
bacterioid, bacteroid	resembling bacteria
balance	1) an apparatus for weighing; 2) the normal state of action between organs
balanus	glans penis
Ballance	eponym: Ballance, Sir Charles A., English physician, 1856-1936. Ballance sign
bleb	a large flaccid vesicle
bled	past tense of bleed
brachial	relating to the arm
branchial	relating to the gills
bronchial	relating to the bronchi
bronchiole	one of approximately six generations of increasingly finer subdivisions of the bronchi
branny	small husklike scales, used in reference to skin flakes
brawny	thickened and dusky, as of a swelling
cancra	plural of cancrum
chancre	the primary lesion of syphilis
carbaril	a cholinesterase inhibitor used as a parasiticide
carbaryl	a cholinesterase-inhibiting contact insecticide
carbonyl	the characteristic group of the ketones, aldehydes, and organic acids
caries	dental decay
carries	harbors an infectious agent or disease

Term	Meaning
carissin	a glucoside obtained from the *Carissa ovata stolonifera* of Australia; a powerful cardiac
carnosine	*N*-β-Alanyl-L-histidine; the dominant nonprotein nitrogenous component of brain tissue
Carrasyn	a wound dressing
Carman	eponym: Carman, Russell D., U.S. radiologist, 1875-1926. Carman sign
carmine	red coloring matter used as a histology stain
corpsman	an enlisted military person who is trained to provide basic medical care
Karmen	eponym: Karmen, Albert, U.S. internist and clinical pathologist, born in 1930. Karmen unit
carotid	an artery
parotid	a gland
Carrion	eponym: Carrion, Daniel A., Peruvian medical student, 1859-1885, Carrion disease
kerion	a granulomatous secondarily infected lesion complicating fungal infection of the hair
catalepsy	a condition characterized by waxy rigidity of the limbs
cataplexy	a transient attack of extreme generalized weakness
cecum	the cul-de-sac lying below the terminal ileum forming the first part of the large intestine
sebum	secretion of the sebaceous glands

Term	Meaning
chalcosis	chronic copper poisoning
chalicosis	pneumoconiosis caused by inhaling dust incident to the occupation of stone cutting
chloroform	formerly used as an inhaled general anesthesia; may be used as a solvent
choleriform	resembling cholera
choreiform	synonym: choroids. The middle vascular tunic of the eye lying between the pigment epithelium and the sclera
chord	1) the simultaneous sound of three or more pitches; 2) a segment of line that brings two points together on a curve
chorda	a tendinous or a cordlike structure
cord	in anatomy, any ropelike structure
chorea	spasmodic, involuntary movements of the limbs or facial muscles
coria	plural of corium
circumcision	an operation to remove part or all of the prepuce
sursumversion	the act of rotating the eyes upward
cirrhonosus	fetal disease that is marked by a yellow staining of the peritoneum and pleura
cirrhosis	endstage liver disease
cirrhotic	relating to or affected with cirrhosis or advanced fibrosis
psychotic	relating to or affected by psychosis
saccadic	quick movement of the eyes

Term	Meaning
CNS	abbreviation: central nervous system
C&S	abbreviation: culture and sensitivity
colicin	bacteriocin produced by strains of E. coli and other enterobacteria
collacin	degenerated collagen
collum	alternate word for neck
column	an anatomic part or structure in the form of a pillar or cylindric funiculus
conjugant	a member of a mating pair of organisms or gametes undergoing conjugation
conjugate	joined or paired
cremation	the process of incinerating a corpse
crenation	the process of becoming a shriveled red blood cell
cruor	coagulated blood
crura	plural of crus
curare	an extract of various plants
cuspad	in a direction toward the cuspid of a tooth
cuspid	having only one cusp
cyst	an abnormal sac that contains a semisolid material and has a membranous lining
sitz	a type of bath
decimate	to kill or destroy
desiccate	to dry thoroughly
desquamate	to shred, peel, or scale off
defenses	the psychological mechanisms used to control anxiety
defensins	a class of basic antibiotic polypeptides that kills bacteria by causing membrane damage

Term	Meaning
deflection	1) moving to one side; 2) in an EKG, a deviation of the curve from the isoelectric base line
deflexion	describes the position of the fetal head in relation to the maternal pelvis in which the head Is descending in a nonflexed attitude
diaphysis	an elongated rodlike structure, as part of a long bone between the epiphysial extremities
diathesis	the constitutional or inborn state disposing to a disease or metabolic or structural anomaly
Ebstein	eponym: Ebstein, Wilhelm, German physician, 1836-1912. Ebstein anomaly, disease, sign
Epstein	eponym: Epstein, Michael Anthony, English virologist, died 1921. Epstein-Barr virus
Epstein	Eponym: Alois, German pediatrician, 1849-1918. Epstein disease, pearls
ectal	outer, external
ictal	relating to or caused by a stroke or seizure
eczema	inflammatory conditions of the skin
exemia	a condition in which a portion of the blood is removed from main circulation but remains within blood vessels
embole	reduction of a limb dislocation
emboli	plural of embolus

Term	Meaning
enterocele	a hernial protrusion through a defect in the rectovaginal or vesicovaginal pouch
entocele	an internal hernia
epidermal	relating to the epidermis
epidural	upon the dura mater
epineural	on the neural arch of a vertebra
ethanal	synonym: acetaldehyde
ethanol	synonym: alcohol
ethenyl	synonym: vinyl
ethinyl	synonym: ethynyl
ethynyl	a monovalent radical. synonym: acetenyl; ethinyl
facial	relating to the face
fascial	relating to any fascia
faucial	relating to the fauces
fascicle	a band or bundle of fibers
vesical	relating to any bladder
vesicle	a small, circumscribed elevation of the skin that contains fluid
fascicular	relating to a fasciculus
vesicular	relating to a vesicle
fissula	a small fissure or cleft
fistula	an abnormal passage from one epithelial surface to another epithelial surface
foreskin	term for prepuce
forskolin	a phorbol ester that binds to and activates protein kinase C

Term	Meaning
formin	a family of proteins that participates in cell polarization, cytokinesis, and vertebrate limb formation
forming	a form in process
fovea	any natural depression on the surface of the body
phoria	relative directions assumed by the eyes during binocular fixation of a given object in the absence of an adequate fusion stimulus
gait	manner of walking
gate	to close an ion channel by electrical or chemical action
globus	a round body
glomus	a small globular body
glucose	dextrose
gulose	one of eight pairs of aldohexoses
heparan	an enzyme
heparin	an anticoagulant principle
homonomous	denoting parts, having similar form and structure, arranged in a series
homonymous	having the same name or expressed in the same terms
human	*Homo sapien*; a person
humin	an insoluble brownish or blackish residue obtained upon acid hydrolysis of glycoproteins
humerus	a bone of the arm
humorous	amusing; funny
hyalin	an eosinophilic homogeneous substance occurring in cellular degeneration
hyaline	relating to clear or colorless fungal structures

Term	Meaning
hypothermia	a body temperature significantly less than 98.6°F
hypothymia	depression of spirits
ichorous	relating to thin watery discharge from an ulcer or unhealthy wound
icterus	synonym: jaundice
ictus	a stroke or attack
ileac	relating to the ileus (obstruction of the intestine)
iliac	relating to the ilium (hip bone)
iniac	relating to the inion (a point located on the external occipital protuberance)
keratorus	vaultlike corneal herniation with severe regular myopic astigmatism
keratosis	any lesion on the epidermis marked by the presence of circumscribed overgrowths of the horny layer
ketamine	a parenterally administered anesthetic that produces catatonia, profound analgesia, increased sympathetic activity and little relaxation of skeletal muscles
ketimine	a tautomer of an aldimine
ketene	a highly reactive acetylating agent, used in chemical syntheses
ketone	any organic compound in which two carbon atoms are linked by the carbon of a carbonyl group
ketose	a carbohydrate containing the characteristic carbonyl group of the ketones
ketosis	a condition characterized by the enhanced production of ketone bodies

Term	Meaning
Korotkoff	eponym: Korotkoff, Nikolai, Russian physician, 1874-1920. Korotkoff sounds, test
Korsakoff	eponym: Korsakoff, Sergei S., Russian neurologist and psychiatrist, 1853-1900. Korsakoff psychosis, syndrome
limbus	the edge, border, or fringe of a part
lumbus	synonym: loin
loop	a sharp curve or bend in a vessel or cord
loupe	a magnifying lens
lues	syphilis
Luys	eponym: Luys, Jules Bernard, French physician, 1828-1897. Luys body
malar	relating to the cheek or cheekbones
molar	1) denoting a grinding, abrading, or wearing away; 2) molar tooth; 3) massive; relating to a mass; not molecular
medial lemniscus	a band of white fibers originating from the gracile and cuneate nuclei and decussating in the lower medulla
medial meniscus	crescent-shaped intraarticular cartilage of the knee joint attached to the medial border of the upper articular surface of the tibia occupying the space surrounding the contacting surfaces of the femur and tibia
meiosis	a special process of cell division comprising two nuclear divisions in rapid succession that result in four gametocytes
miosis	contraction of the pupil of the eye

Term	Meaning
menthane	the monocyclic terpene parent of alcohols
methane	an odorless gas produced by the decomposition of organic matter
methene	an odorless gas produced by the decomposition of organic matter
mica	a group of aluminum silicate minerals
mika	mika operation: the establishment of a permanent fistula in the bulbous portion of the urethra to render the man incapable of procreating
morpheme	the smallest linguistic unit with a meaning
morphine	a narcotic used for pain control
mucase	synonym: mucinase
mucous	relating to mucous
mucus	clear viscid secretion of the mucous membranes
myotome	a knife for dividing muscle
myotone	synonym: myotony; muscular tonus or tension
narcosis	general and nonspecific reversible depression of neuronal excitability
necrosis	pathological death of one or more cells
necrotic	pertaining to or affected by necrosis
nephrotic	relating to, caused by, or similar to nephrosis
neuralgic	relating to, resembling, or of the character of neuralgia
neurologic	relating to neurology

Term	Meaning
neutron	an electrical neutral particle in the nuclei of all atoms with a mass slightly larger than a proton
nitron	a reagent for the determination of nitric acid
nervous	1) relating to a nerve or nerves; 2) easily agitated
nervus	(L.) nerves
nevus	a circumscribed malformation of the skin
nitride	a compound of nitrogen and one other element
nitrite	a salt of nitrous acid
nodal	referring to a node
notal	referring to the back
notation	to make a note
nutation	the act of nodding, especially involuntary nodding
oscillation	a to-and-fro movement
oscitation	synonym: yawning
osmesis	synonym: olfaction
osmosis	the process by which solvent tends to move through a semipermeable that will hold back the solutes
osteal	synonym: osseous
ostial	relating to any orifice, or ostium
osteopetrosis	excessive formation of dense trabecular bone and calcified cartilage
osteoporosis	reduction in the quantity of bone or atrophy of skeletal tissue
paler	more pale
pallor	paleness, as of the skin

Term	Meaning
parenteral	by some other means other than through the gastrointestinal tract
parietal	relating to the wall of any cavity
preretinal	anterior to the retina
pecten	a structure with comblike processes or projections
pectin	gastrointestinal absorbent medication
pediatrics	the medical speciality concerned with the study of children in health and disease from birth through adolescence
podiatrics	the medical speciality concerned with the study of the human feet
perfusion	the flow of blood per unit volume of tissue
profusion	a score reflecting the number of visible lesions in a region on chest radiograph of an individual with pneumoconiosis
perineal	referring to the perineum
peroneal	synonym: fibular
phthalic	phthalic acid
thallic	related to thallium
physic	1) the art of medicine; 2) a medicine
Physick	eponym: Physick, Philip Syng, U.S. surgeon, 1768-1837. Physick pouches
physique	the physical or bodily structure
pica	a perverted appetite for substances not fit as food, or of no nutritional value
plica	synonym: fold
pleuritis	inflammation of the pleura
pruritus	itching

Term	Meaning
portable	capable of being easily moved
potable	fit to drink
postnasal	posterior to the nasal cavity
postnatal	occurring after birth
posttraumatic	occurring after trauma and, by implication, caused by it
posttrematic	relating to the caudal surface of the branchial cleft
proband	in human genetics, the patient or family member who brings a family under study
probang	a flexible rod used to try to advance or retrieve foreign bodies from the esophagus, considered to be dangerous
psychosis	a mental and behavioral disorder that causes distortion of one's mental capacity
sycosis	a pustular folliculitis
radicular	1) relating to a radicle; 2) pertaining to the root of a tooth
reticular	relating to a reticulum
refection	restoring to normal state
reflection	in psychotherapy, a technique in which a patient's statements are repeated, restated, or rephrased so that the patient will continue to explore and expound on emotionally significant content
reflex	an involuntary reaction in response to a stimulus
reflux	a backward flow, regurgitation
retinal	relating to the eye's retina
retinol	a half-carotene

Term	Meaning
salute	to recognize with a gesture prescribed by regulation
solute	the dissolved substance in a solution
Schilder disease	1) diffuse sclerosis or encephalitis periaxialis diffusa; 2) the leukodystrophies
Schindler disease	an autosomal recessive disorder
scleredema	hard, nonpitting edema of the skin
scleroderma	thickening and induration of the skin caused by new collagen formation
xeroderma	a mild form of ichthyosis
scutum	1) synonym: scute; 2) a plate in ixodid ticks
sputum	expectorated matter
selectin	a cell surface molecule involved in immune adhesion and cell trafficking
selection	the combined effect of the causes and consequences of genetic factors
serene	calm
serine	the L-isomer is one of the amino acids in proteins
skin graft	a piece of skin transplanted from one part of the body to another
syngraft	a tissue or organ transplanted from one member of a species to another genetically identical member
stent	a thread, needle, or catheter, lying within the lumen of tubular structures
Stent	eponym: Stent, Charles R., English dentist, died 1901. Stent graft

Term	Meaning
stoop	1) to bend far forward; 2) a small porch
stupe	a cloth wrung out of hot water, usually impregnated with an irritant to produce counterirritation
stroma	the framework of an organ, gland, or other structure
struma	1) synonym: goiter; 2) formerly, any enlargement of a tissue
tabid	synonym: tabetic; progressive wasting or emaciation
tepid	lukewarm
tache	a circumscribed discoloration of the skin or mucous membrane
cache	hidden
taction	the sense of touch
traction	the act of drawing or pulling
taenia	a coiled, bandlike anatomic structure
tinea	a fungal infection of the keratin component of the hair, skin, or nails
thein	synonym: caffeine
thenen	relating only to the palm
transverse	crosswise
traverse	in computed tomography, one complete linear movement of the gantry across the object being scanned
trehalase	a glycosidase secreted in the duodenum
trehalose	a nonreducing disaccharide
varicose	relating to, affected by, or characterized by varices
verrucose, verrucous	resembling a wart

Term	Meaning
varies	changes; alterations
Veress	eponym: Veress, Janos, Hungarian physician. Veress needle
Voorhees	eponym: origin unknown. Voorhees needle
Voorhoeve	eponym: Voorhoeve, N., Dutch radiologist, 1879-1927. Voorhoeve disease
varix	a dilated vein
varus	bent or twisted toward the midline of the limb or body
venose	having veins
venous	relating to a vein
vertex	1) in craniometry, the topmost point of the vault of the skull; 2) in obstetrics, a portion of the fetal head
vortex	synonym: 1) verticil; 2) whorl
vesicostomy	synonym: cystostomy
viscosity	the resistance to flow or alteration of shape by any substance as a result of molecular cohesion
wan	extremely pale
wen	a cyst

Spanish-English Medical Phrases

Overview of Spanish Pronunciation

Spanish letter(s)	Equivalent English sound (in italics)
a	Similar to f*a*ther
b	Similar to a*b*normal
c	Hard when it precedes a, o, or u (similar to es*c*ape); soft when it precedes e or i (similar to pa*c*e)
ch	Similar to *ch*ild
cu	Similar to *qu*estion
d	Similar to *d*ay when it begins a word; similar to wi*th* in the middle or end of a word
e	Similar to s*e*psis; the Spanish "e" does not end with the glide of the English ey as in th*ey*
f	Similar to per*f*orate
g	Similar to *g*out when it precedes a, o, u, or a consonant; similar to *h*ospital when it precedes e or i
h	Always silent
i	Similar to s*ee*
j	Similar to *h*ospital
k	Similar to ma*k*e
l	Similar to s*l*eep
ll	Similar to mi*lli*on
m	Similar to ato*m*ic
n	Similar to co*m*ma when it precedes b, p, or v; silent when it precedes m; otherwise similar to lear*n*ing
ñ	Similar to o*ni*on

Spanish letter(s)	Equivalent English sound (in italics)
o	Similar to l**o**w
p	Similar to **sp**it
q	Similar to **k**ey
r	Similar to hai**r**y
rr	Always trilled. Words spelled with one "r" have a different meaning than those spelled with two. For example: • *pero* (but) and *perro* (dog) • *caro* (expensive) and *carro* (wagon, cart, car) • *para* (for) and *parra* (grapevine)
s	Similar to ba**s**ement
t	Similar to s**t**ent
u	Similar to fl**u**
v	Same as the Spanish b; similar to sa**b**le
x	Similar to me**ss**age when it precedes a consonant; otherwise similar to fle**x**
y	Similar to bo**y**; when meaning "and," similar to s**ee**
z	Similar to **c**ity

Spanish vowels are almost always pronounced the same as English vowels. They are short, tense, and neither drawn out or glided.

There are two categories of Spanish vowels: strong vowels (a, e, and o) and weak vowels (i and u). A combination of a strong and a weak vowel or two weak vowels is pronounced as a single syllable, forming a diphthong (an unsegmented gliding sound in which the weak sounds [i and u] are barely audible), such as in *lengua*, *nueve*, and *biopsia*. A written accent over the weak vowel breaks the diphthong and forms two separate syllables, such as in *día* and *sangría*.

The meaning of a word can change with the addition of a written accent. For example:

• *Seria* (serious) versus *sería* (would be)

• *Continuo* (continuous) and *continuó* (he continued)

• *Papa* (potato, especially in Latin America) and *papá* (father)

For more information and audio pronunciations, please refer to the CD that accompanies this book.

Spanish Phrases

English	Spanish
Emergency Response	
Do you have difficulty speaking?	¿Tiene usted dificultad en hablar?
Are you having any pain?	¿Tiene usted dolor actualmente?
Where is the pain?	¿Dónde le duele?
Can you point to the area where you feel pain?	¿Me puede indicar donde siente usted el dolor?
Do you ever have chest pain or discomfort?	¿Alguna vez tiene usted dolor de pecho o molestia?
Have you ever had an allergic reaction to a medication?	¿Ha tenido usted alguna vez una reacción alérgica a algún medicamento?

English	Spanish

Medication Phrases

English	Spanish
I would like to give you:	Quisiera darle a usted un(a):
an injection	inyección
an intravenous medication	medicamento por vía intrvenosa
a liquid medication	medicamento en forma líquida
a medicated cream or powder	medicamento en pomada o polvo
a medication through your epidural catheter	medicamento por el catéter epidural
a medication through your rectum	medicamento por el recto
a medication through your ____tube	medicamento por su ___tubo
a medication under your tongue	medicamento debajo de la lengua
your pill(s)	su(s) píldora(s)
a suppository	supositorio

English	Spanish
This medication will:	Este medicamento hará que:
elevate your blood pressure	su presión sanguínea suba
improve circulation to your _____.	la circulación por ___ mejore
lower your blood pressure	su presión anguínea baje
lower your blood sugar	el nivel de azúcar en la sangre baje
make your heart rhythm more even	el ritmo del corazón sea más uniforme

English	Spanish
raise your blood sugar	su nivel de azúcar en la sange suba
reduce or prevent the formation of blood clots	se reduzca o evite la formación de coágulos de sangre
remove fluid from your body	se le quite fluido del cuerpo
remove fluid from your feet, ankles, or legs	se le quite fluido de los pies, tobillos, o piernas
remove fluid from your lungs so that they work better	se le quite fluido de los pulmones para que funcionen mejor
remove fluid from your pancreas so that it works better	se le quite fluido del páncreas para que funcione mejor
This medication will help your body to:	Este medicamento le ayudará a su cuerpo a:
kill the bacteria in your___	destruir la bacteria de la (región infectada)
slow down your heart rate	reducir el latido cardiaco
soften your bowel movements	ablandar sus evacuaciones
speed up your heart rate	acelerar el latido cardiaco
use insulin more efficiently	usar la insulina más eficazmente
This medication will help you to:	Este medicamento le ayudará a usted a:
breathe better	respirar con mayor facilidad
fight infections	luchar contra infecciones

English	Spanish
relax	relajarse
sleep	dormir
think more clearly	pensar con mayor claridad
This medication will relieve or reduce:	Este medicamento le aliviará o disminuirá:
the acid production in your stomach	la producción de ácido en el estómago
anxiety	la angustia
bladder spasms	los espasmos en la vejiga
burning in your stomach or chest	la sensación ardiente en el estómago o tórax
burning when you urinate	la sensación ardiente al orinar
diarrhea	la diarrea
muscle cramps	los espasmos musculares
nausea	las náuseas
pain in your_____	el dolor en la (el)_____
This medication will help your body to produce more or less:	Este medicamento ayudará a su cuerpo a producir más o menos:
antibodies	anticuerpos
clotting factors	factores o agenres coagulantes
insulin	insulina
platelets	plaquetas
red blood cells	glóbulos rojos
white blood cells	glóbulos blancos
This medication or treatment will destroy:	Este medicamento o tratamiento destruirá:
bacteria	bacterias
cancer cells	células cancerosas

English	Spanish
Commonly Used	
Hello	Hola
Good morning	Buenos días
Good afternoon	Buenas tardes
Good evening	Buenas noches
Come in please.	Pase usted por favor.
My name is _____.	Me llamo_____.
Who is the patient?	¿Quién es el (la) paciente?
What is your name?	¿Cómo se llama usted?
It is nice to meet you.	Mucho gusto en conocerle.
How are you?	¿Cómo está usted?
I need you to sign this form.	Necesito que usted firme este formulario.
Please	Por favor
Thank you	Gracias
Yes	Sí
No	No
Maybe	Quizás or tal vez
Sometimes	A veces
How are you feeling?	¿Cómo se siente usted?
What time is it?	¿Qué hora es?
What day is it?	¿Qué día es hoy?
What is the date?	¿A qué fecha estamos?
Where are you?	¿Dónde está usted?
How old are you?	¿Cuántos años tiene usted?
Did you come alone?	¿Vino usted solo(a)?
Who brought you?	¿Quién le trajo?
Where were you born?	¿Dónde nació usted?
Where do you live?	¿Dónde vive usted?
What is your address?	¿Cuál es su dirección?
Do you live alone?	¿Vive usted solo(a)?

English	Spanish
Who lives with you?	¿Quién vive con usted?
Are you:	¿Es usted:
single?	¿soltero(a)?
married?	¿casado(a)?
divorced?	¿divordiado(a)?
widowed?	¿viudo(a)?
separated?	¿(Esta usted) separado(a)?
Do you have any children?	¿Tiene usted hijos?
Did you go to school?	¿Asistió usted a la escuela?
Where do you work?	¿Dónde trabaja usted?
What is your religion?	¿Cuál es su religión?

General Instructions

Bend over backward.	Inclínese usted hacia atrás.
Bend over forward.	Inclínese usted hacia adelante.
Don't talk.	No hable usted.
Lean backward.	Recuéstese usted.
Lean forward.	Inclínese usted hacia adelante.
Lie down.	Acuéstese usted.
Lie on your:	Acuéstese usted de:
back	boca arriba
left side	lado izquierdo
right side	lado derecho
stomach	boca abajo
Roll over.	Dé usted una vuelta.
Say "ahhhh."	Diga usted "aaaa."

English	Spanish
Sit down.	Siéntese usted.
Sit up.	Enderécese usted.
Stand up.	Póngase usted de pie.
Turn to the side.	Voltéese usted hacia un lado.
Whisper.	Murmure usted.

General Teaching

I'm going to take your vital signs.	Voy a tomarle a usted los signos vitales.
Blood pressure	La presión sanguinea
Pulse	El pulso
Respirations	La respiración
Temperature	La temperatura
I'm going to take a blood sample.	Voy a tomarle a usted una muestra de sangre.
You need to provide a urine specimen.	Tiene usted que darnos un espécimen de orina.
Are you comfortable?	¿Está usted confortable?
Does this hurt?	¿Le duele a usted esto?
Where does it hurt?	¿Dónde le duele a usted?
Let me show you how to do it.	Permítame enseñarle cómo hacerlo.
Let's practice together.	Vamos a ensayar junto(a) s.
I want you to do it yourself.	Quiero que usted to haga por sí solo(a).

English	Spanish
I will watch to make sure you do it correctly.	Le observaré para estar seguro(a) de que usted lo puede hacer por sí solo(a).
Let me know if you have trouble.	Dígame si usted tiene dificultad en.
You'll need to walk with a cane.	Usted necesitará andr con bastón.
You'll need to use a walker.	Usted necesitará usar un andador.

Personal Care

Bedpan	Basín plano
Here is a bedpan if you need to:	Aquí tiene una cuña por si usted tiene que:
move your bowels	evacuar
urinate	orinar
Do you need to use the bedpan?	¿Necesita usted usar la cuña?
Call me when you're finished with the bedpan.	Llámeme cuando acabe de usar la cuña.
Bedside commode	Silla retrete al lado de la cama
You can't walk to the bathroom.	Usted no puede caminar al baño.
I can get you a bedside commode.	Le puedo traer una silla retrete.

English	Spanish
Call me when you're finished using the commode.	Llámeme cuando haya acabado de usar la silla retrete.
Blanket	Cobija
Do you need a blanket?	¿Necesita usted una manta (cobija)?
Emesis basin	Phalangana para vómitos
This is an emesis basin.	Aquí está una cubeta para vómito.
You can use the emesis basin if you need to vomit.	Usted puede usar esta cubeta si tiene que vomitar.
Enema	Enema
This is an enema.	Éste es un enema.
You need an enema to help you move your bowels.	Usted necesita un enema (lavativo) para ayudarle a evacuar.
Lie on your left side.	Acuéstese del lado izquierdo.
I'm going to put this tube in your rectum.	Voy a insertarle este tubo en el recto.
Take a deep breath.	Respire usted profundamente.
Let me know if you experience any cramping.	Dígame por favor si siente retortijones.
Try to retain the fluid.	Trate usted de retener el liquido.
Oral care	Cuidado oral
How do you care for your teeth and gums?	¿Qué cuidado da usted a los dientes y las encías?
Toothbrush	Cepillo de dientes
Toothpaste	Pasta de dientes

English	Spanish
Urinal	Orinal
Here is a urinal.	Aquí está un orinal.
Do you need to use the urinal?	¿Necesita usted usar el orinal?
Call me when you're finished with the urinal.	Llámeme cuando acabe de usar el orinal.
Wash basin	Cubeta lava
I'll get you a basin to wash yourself.	Le voy a traer una cubeta para que se lave usted.
Call me when you're finished with the basin.	Llámeme cuando haya acabado de usar la cubeta.

Nutrition

Dietary influences	Influencias en la dieta
Does your ethnic or cultural background influence your diet?	¿Su origen étnico o cultural ejerce una influencia sobre su dieta?
How does it influence it?	¿Cómo la influye?
Do you just eat vegetables?	¿Come usted sólo verduras?
Do you eat red meat?	¿Come usted carne roja?
Do you just eat chicken or fish?	¿Come usted sólo pollo o pescado?
Does your religion restrict or otherwise affect what you eat?	¿Su religión limita o de cualquier modo afecta lo que usted come?
How?	¿Cómo lo afecta?
Do you fast or not eat food on any special days?	¿Ayuna usted o no come nada durante días especiales?

English	Spanish
Do you not eat meat on Fridays?	¿No come usted carne los viernes?
Weight	Peso
Have you gained any weight recently?	¿Ha aumentado de peao últimamente?
Have you lost any weight recently?	¿Ha bajado usted de peso últimamente?
How much?	¿Cuánto?
Fluid intake	Toma de fluidos
How much fluid do you drink during the day?	¿Cuánto líquido bebe usted al día?
Special diets	Dietas especiales
Do you follow a special diet?	¿Tiene usted una dieta especial?
What kind of diet?	¿Qué clase de dieta?
How long have you been on the diet?	¿Hace cuánto a usted la dieta?
What is the reason for the diet?	¿Cuánto tiempo que tiene usted esta dieta?
How much salt do you use, if any?	¿Cuánta sal usa usted, si es que la usa?
You need to reduce salt in your diet.	Usted necesita reducir el contenido de sal en su dieta.
Avoid adding salt:	Evite usted añadir sal:
while cooking your food	cuando cocine su comida
to your meals at the table	a su comida en la mesa
You need to reduce cholesterol in your diet.	Usted necesita reducir el colesterol en su dieta.
Some foods that you shouldn't eat are:	Algunos de los alimentos que usted no debe comer son:
butter	mantequilla

English	Spanish
shortening	grasa (manteca)
egg yolks	yemas de huevo
biscuits	panecillos
cheese	queso
avocados	aguacate
bacon	tocino
sausage	salchicha
hot dogs	perros calientes
shellfish	mariscos
ice cream	helado
chocolate	chocolate
liver	higado
most red meat	la mayoría de la carne roja
You need to add fiber to your diet.	Usted tiene que añadir fibra a su dieta.
Eat fresh fruit and vegetables.	Coma usted fruta fresca y verduras.
Some high-fiber fruits include apples, oranges, and peaches.	Algunas frutas de alta fibra incluyen las manzanas, naranjas y melocotones.
Some high-fiber vegetables include carrots, string beans, broccoli, and peas.	Algunas verduras que contienen alta fibra incluyen las zanahorias, ejotes, brécol y guisantes (chícharos).
Eat whole grain breads, such as whole wheat and pumpernickel, and whole grain cereals, such as bran flakes, oat flakes, oatmeal, and shredded wheat.	Coma pan integral, como pan de trigo entero y pan negro de centeno, y cereal de grano integral, coma hojuelas de avena, harina de avena y trigo molido.
Add unprocessed bran to your food.	Añada salvado de trigo sin procesar a sus comidas.

Eat dried peas and beans, such as lentils, and navy, kidney, or pinto beans.	Coma usted guisantes secos y frijoles comolentejas, frijoles rojos, frijoles negros y frioles pintos.
Remember to drink at least six 8-ounce glasses of fluid per day.	No se olvide usted de tomar por lo menos seis vasos de ocho onzas de líquido al día.

Adapted from McElroy OH, Grabb LL. *Spanish-English, English-Spanish Medical Dictionary*, 3rd ed. Baltimore: Lippincott Williams & Wilkins, 2005 and *English & Spanish Medical Words & Phrases*, 3rd ed. Springhouse, PA: Lippincott Williams & Wilkins, 2004.

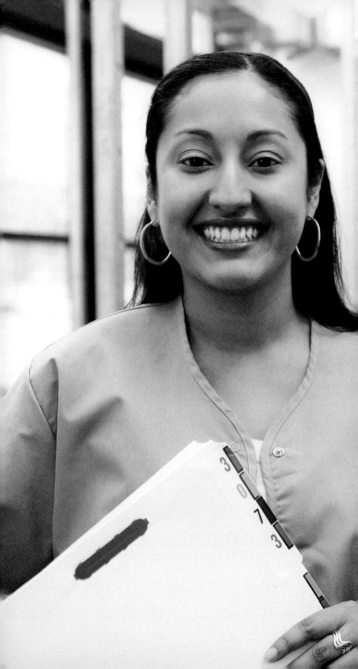

Abbreviations, Acronyms, and Symbols

Abbreviations and Acronyms

Abbreviation/ Acronym	Meaning
α	alpha: Bunsen solubility coefficient; first in a series; specific rotation term; heavy chain class corresponding to IgA
$\bar{a}$	before
a	specific absorption coefficient (usually italic); total acidity; area; systemic arterial blood (subscript); asymmetric; atto-
A	adenosine (or adenylic acid); alveolar gas (subscript); ampere; anterior; assessment
Ab	antibody; abortion
ABG	arterial blood gas
ABO	blood group system
ABO-Rh	ABO blood group, rhesus antigen
ABR	abortus-Bang-ring (test); auditory brainstem response (audiometry)
ABVD	Adriamycin (doxorubicin), bleomycin, vinblastine, and dacarbazine
AC	acetate; acromioclavicular; atriocarotid
a.c.	[L.] *ante cibum* or *ante cibos,* before a meal
ACE *(ās)*	angiotensin-converting enzyme

Abbreviation/ Acronym	Meaning
ACS	acute coronary syndrome
ACT	activated coagulation time
AD	[L.] *auris dextra*, right ear; Alzheimer disease
ADA	Americans with Disabilities Act
ADH	antidiuretic hormone; alcohol dehydrogenase
ADL	activities of daily living
ad lib.	[L.] *ad libitum*, freely, as desired
ADH	antidiuretic hormone
ADHD	attention-deficit/hyperactivity disorder
AED	automated external defibrillator
Ag	antigen; [L.] *argentum*, silver
AID	artificial insemination donor
AIDS *(ādz)*	acquired immunodeficiency syndrome
AIH	artificial insemination by husband; artificial insemination, homologous
AJCCS	American Joint Committee on Cancer Staging (criteria)
AKA	above-knee amputation
Al	aluminum
alb	albumin
ALL	acute lymphocytic leukemia
ALS	amyotrophic lateral sclerosis
ALT	alanine aminotransferase (enzyme)
a.m.	morning
AMA	antimitochondrial antibody
AML	acute myelogenous leukemia
amt	amount
Amu	atomic mass unit
ANA	antinuclear antibody
ANS	autonomic nervous system

Abbreviation/ Acronym	Meaning
AP	anterior-posterior
A&P	auscultation and percussion
APAP	acetaminophen
Apgar *(ap'gär)*	appearance, pulse, grimace, activity, respiration
aq	water
ARF	acute renal failure; acute rheumatic fever
As	arsenic
AS	[L.] *auris sinistra*, left ear
ASA	acetylsalicylic acid (aspirin); antisperm antibodies
ASD	atrial septal defect
ASHD	arteriosclerotic heart disease
AST	aspartate aminotransferase (enzyme)
ATP	adenosine 5'-triphosphate
at. wt.	atomic weight
Au	[L.] *aurum*, gold
AU	[L.] *auris utraque*, each ear, both ears
AV	arteriovenous
A-V	arteriovenous; atrioventricular
AVN	atrioventricular node
AW	atomic weight
A&W	alive and well
ax.	axis
β	second in a series; blood (subscript)
b	blood (subscript)
B	barometric pressure (subscript); boron
Ⓑ	bilateral
Ba	barium
BADL	basic activities of daily living
BAEP	brainstem auditory evoked potential
BAER	brainstem auditory evoked response

Abbreviation/ Acronym	Meaning
BBB	blood-brain barrier
BE	barium enema
B-E	below-the-elbow amputation
BCC	basal cell carcinoma
BD	bipolar disorder
Bi	bismuth
b.i.d.	[L.] *bis in die*, twice a day
BIPAP	bilevel positive airway pressure
BKA	below-knee amputation
BM	bowel movement
BMI	body mass index
BMP	basic metabolic panel (chem-7, SMA-7)
BP	blood pressure; boiling point; British Pharmacopoeia
BPH	benign prostatic hyperplasia
Br	bromine
BRAT	diet of banana, rice cereal, applesauce, toast
BRCA	breast cancer antigen
BRP	bathroom privileges
BS	blood sugar
BSA	body surface area
BT	bleeding time
BTU	British thermal unit
BUN	blood urea nitrogen
BUN:Cr	blood urea nitrogen to creatinine ratio
Bx	biopsy
$\bar{c}$	with
C	calorie (large); carbon; Celsius; centigrade; clearance rate, renal (as subscript); compliance; concentration; cylindrical lens; cytidine

Abbreviation/ Acronym	Meaning
c	calorie (small); capillary blood (subscript); centi-
ca.	[L.] *circa*, about, approximately
CA	cancer; carcinoma; cardiac arrest; chronologic age; croup-associated (virus); cytosine arabinoside; cancer antigen; carbohydrate antigen
CABG *(ka'bij)*	coronary artery bypass graft
CAD	coronary artery disease
cal	calorie (small)
Cal	calorie (large)
cap	capsule
CAT *(kat)*	computerized axial tomography
CBC	complete blood (cell) count
cc, c.c.	cubic centimeter
CC	chief complaint
CCK	cholecystokinin
CCU	coronary care unit; critical care unit
Cd	cadmium
C. diff	*Clostridium difficile*
CEA	carcinoembryonic antigen
CF	complement fixation; cystic fibrosis; coupling factor
CH, CHF	congestive heart failure
CHO	carbohydrate
CI	color index
CIB	[L.] *cibus*, food
CIS	carcinoma in situ
CJD	Creutzfeldt-Jakob disease
Cl	chlorine
CL	cardiolipin

Abbreviation/ Acronym	Meaning
CLIA	Clinical Laboratory Improvement Amendments
CLL	chronic lymphocytic leukemia
cm	centimeter
Cm	curium
CMC	carpometacarpal
CML	chronic myelogenous leukemia
CMV	controlled mechanical ventilation; cytomegalovirus
CNS	central nervous system
c/o	complains of
Co	cobalt
CO	cardiac output
CO_2	carbon dioxide
CoA	coenzyme A
COG	center of gravity
COPD	chronic obstructive pulmonary disease
CP	cerebral palsy; costophrenic
CPAP (sē'pap)	continuous (or constant) positive airway pressure
CPPB	continuous (or constant) positive-pressure breathing
CPPV	continuous positive-pressure ventilation
CPR	cardiopulmonary resuscitation
cps	cycles per second
Cr	chromium; creatinine
CR	conditioned reflex; crown-rump length
CRD	chronic respiratory disease
CRP	cross-reacting protein
CRST	calcinosis cutis, Raynaud phenomenon, sclerodactyly, and telangiectasia syndrome

Abbreviation/ Acronym	Meaning
C&S	culture and sensitivity
CSD	catscratch disease
CSF	cerebrospinal fluid
CT	computed tomography
CTA	computed tomographic angiography
Cu	[L.] *cuprum*, copper
cu mm, mm^3	cubic millimeter
CV	cardiovascular
CVA	cerebrovascular accident
CVP	central venous pressure
CVS	chorionic villus sampling
CXR	chest x-ray
Cys	cysteine
Cyt	cytosine
Δ	delta; change; heat
d	deci-; day
D	dead space gas (subscript); deciduous; deuterium; diffusing capacity; dihydrouridine (in nucleic acids); diopter; [L.] *dexter,* right (opposite of left); vitamin D potency of cod liver oil
db, dB	decibel
D&C	dilation and curettage
D-dimer	fibrin degradation product
DDS	doctor of dental surgery
D&E	dilation and evacuation
def	decayed, extracted, or filled (deciduous teeth)
DEF	decayed, extracted, or filled (permanent teeth)
df	decayed and filled (deciduous teeth)
DF	decayed and filled (permanent teeth)

Abbreviation/ Acronym	Meaning
DJD	degenerative joint disease
DKA	diabetic ketoacidosis
DMD	Duchenne muscular dystrophy
dmf	decayed, missing, or filled (deciduous teeth)
DMF	decayed, missing, or filled (permanent teeth)
DNA	deoxyribonucleic acid
DNR	do not resuscitate
DOA	dead on arrival
DPI	dry powder inhaler
DPT	dipropyltryptamine; diphtheria, pertussis, and tetanus (vaccines)
dr	dram
DRE	digital rectal examination
DRG	diagnosis-related group
DSA	digital subtraction angiography
dsDNA	double-stranded DNA
DT	delirium tremens; duration of tetany
DTP	diphtheria and tetanus toxoids and pertussis vaccine; distal tingling on percussion (Tinel sign)
DTR	deep tendon reflex
DVT	deep vein thrombosis
Dx	diagnosis
E	exa-; extraction ratio
EB, EBV	Epstein-Barr virus
ECF	extracellular fluid
ECG	electrocardiogram
echo	echocardiogram
ECS	electrocerebral silence
ECT	electroconvulsive therapy

Abbreviation/ Acronym	Meaning
ECU	emergency care unit
ED	effective dose; erectile dysfunction
EDC	estimated date of confinement
EDD	estimated date of delivery
EEG	electroencephalogram
EENT	eye, ear, nose, and throat
EGD	esophagogastroduodenoscopy
eGFR	estimated glomerular filtration rate
EKG	[German] *Elektrokardiogramme*, electrocardiogram
ELISA *(ē-lī'să)*	enzyme-linked immunosorbent assay
EM	electron microscopy
EMC	encephalomyocarditis (virus)
EMS	emergency medical services
ENT	ear, nose, and throat
EP	electrophysiology
EPAP	expiratory positive airway pressure
EPS	electrophysiological study
ER	endoplasmic reticulum; emergency room; estrogen receptor
ERBF	effective renal blood flow
ERV	expiratory reserve volume
ESP	extrasensory perception
ESR	electron spin resonance; erythrocyte sedimentation rate
ESRD	end-stage renal disease
ESWL	extracorporeal shock wave lithotripsy
EtOH, ETOH	ethyl alcohol
EUS	endoscopic ultrasonography
F	Fahrenheit; Faraday constant; fertility factor; field of vision; fluorine; force; fractional concentration; free energy

Abbreviation/ Acronym	Meaning
FB	foreign body
FBS	fasting blood sugar
Fe	[L.] *ferrum*, iron
FEF	forced expiratory flow
FET	forced expiratory time
FEV	forced expiratory volume
FGT	female genital tract
FH	family history
FHR	fetal heart rate
FHT	fetal heart tones
fl oz	fluid ounce
FNA	fine-needle aspiration
FOBT	fecal occult blood test
Fr	francium; French (gauge, scale)
FRC	functional residual capacity (of lungs)
Fru	fructose
FS	frozen section
FSH	follicle-stimulating hormone
FU	fluorouracil
FUO	fever of unknown origin
FVC	forced vital capacity
Fw	F wave (fibrillary wave, flutter wave)
Fx	fracture
γ	gamma; Ostwald solubility coefficient; the third in a series; heavy chain class corresponding to IgG
μg	microgram
g	gram
G	giga-; glucose; Newtonian constant of gravitation; guanosine or guanylic acid residues in polynucleotides; gravida (obstetric history)

Abbreviation/ Acronym	Meaning
Ga	gallium
GAD	generalized anxiety disorder
GC	gonococcus, gonorrhea
GERD *(gĕrd)*	gastroesophageal reflux disease
GFR	glomerular filtration rate
GH	glenohumeral; growth hormone
GI	gastrointestinal; Gingival Index
GIST *(jist)*	gastrointestinal stromal tumor
gm	gram
gr	grain
gt.	[L.] *gutta*, a drop
gtt.	[L.] *guttae*, drops
GTT	glucose tolerance test
GU	genitourinary
GVHD	graft-versus-host disease
Gy	gray (unit of absorbed dose of ionizing radiation)
GYN	gynecology
h	hecto-; hour
H	henry; hydrogen; hyperopia; hyperopic
H^+	hydrogen ion
HAART *(hart)*	highly active antiretroviral therapy
HAV	hepatitis A virus
Hb, Hbg	hemoglobin
HBV	hepatitis B virus
HCG, hCG	human chorionic gonadotropin
HCT, Hct	hematocrit
HCV	hepatitis C virus
HD	Huntington disease
HDL	high-density lipoprotein
He	helium
HEENT	head, eyes, ears, nose, and throat

Abbreviation/ Acronym	Meaning
Hg	[L.] *hydrargyrum*, mercury
HGB, Hgb	hemoglobin
HGH	human (pituitary) growth hormone
H&H	hemoglobin and hematocrit
HHV	human herpes virus
HIPAA *(hip'ă)*	Health Insurance Portability and Accountability Act of 1996
HIV	human immunodeficiency virus
HMO	health maintenance organization
H&P	history and physical
hpf, HPF	high-power field
HPI	history of present illness
HPV	human papilloma virus
H. pylori	*Helicobacter pylori*
HRT	hormone replacement therapy
h. s., HS	[L.] *hora somni*, at bedtime
HSV	herpes simplex virus
HSV-1	herpes simplex virus type 1
HSV-2	herpes simplex virus type 2
Ht	hyperopia, total; height
HTN	hypertension
Hx	medical history
Hz	hertz
I	inspired gas (subscript); iodine
^{123}I	iodine-123 (radioisotope)
^{125}I	iodine-125
^{131}I	iodine-131
IBD	inflammatory bowel disease
IBS	irritable bowel syndrome
ICD	*International Classification of Diseases*; implantable cardioverter defibrillator
ICF	intracellular fluid

Abbreviation/ Acronym	Meaning
ICP	intracranial pressure
ICU	intensive care unit
ID	infective dose; intradermal
I&D	incision and drainage
IF	initiation factor; intrinsic factor
IFN	interferon
Ig	immunoglobulin
IgG	immunoglobulin G
IgM	immunoglobulin M
IH	infectious hepatitis
IL	interleukin
IM	internal medicine; intramuscular(ly); infectious mononucleosis
INR	International Normalized Ratio (prothrombin time)
I&O	(fluid) intake and output
IP	interphalangeal; intraperitoneal(ly); inpatient
IPAP	inspiratory positive airway pressure
IPPV	intermittent positive-pressure ventilation
IPV	inactivated poliovirus vaccine
IQ	intelligence quotient
Ir	iridium
ITP	idiopathic thrombocytopenic purpura; inosine 5′-triphosphate
IU	International Unit
IUCD	intrauterine contraceptive device
IUD	intrauterine device
IV	intravenous, intravenously; intraventricular
IVP	intravenous pyelogram
IVU	intravenous urogram

Abbreviation/ Acronym	Meaning
J	joule
k	kilo-
K	[Modern L.] *kalium*, potassium; kelvin
kcal	kilocalorie
kg	kilogram
KJ	knee jerk
KS	Kaposi sarcoma
KUB	kidneys, ureters, bladder
kv	kilovolt
l	liter
L	inductance; left; [L.] *limes*, boundary, limit; liter
Ⓛ	left
LA	lupus antibody, lupus anticoagulant
LASER *(lā'zĕr)*	light amplification by stimulated emission of radiation
LASIK *(lā'sik)*	laser *in situ* keratomileusis
lb	pound
LBT	lupus band test
LC	lethal concentration
LD	lethal dose
LDL	low-density lipoprotein
LE	left eye; lupus erythematosus
LEEP *(lēp)*	loop electrosurgical excision procedure
LFA	left frontoanterior (fetal position)
LFP	left frontoposterior (fetal position)
LFT	left frontotransverse (fetal position)
LH	luteinizing hormone
Li	lithium
LLQ	left lower quadrant
LMA	left mentoanterior (fetal position)
LMP	left mentoposterior (fetal position)

Abbreviation/ Acronym	Meaning
LMT	left mentotransverse (fetal position)
LOA	left occipitoanterior (fetal position)
LOP	left occipitoposterior (fetal position)
LOT	left occipitotransverse (fetal position)
LP	lumbar puncture
lpf, LPF	low-power field
Lr	lawrencium
LSA	left sacroanterior (fetal position)
LSP	left sacroposterior (fetal position)
LST	left sacrotransverse (fetal position)
LTB	laryngotracheobronchitis
LTH	luteotropic hormone
LTM	long-term memory
LUQ	left upper quadrant
LVET	left ventricular ejection time
LVH	left ventricular hypertrophy
L&W	living and well
lytes	electrolytes
μ	mu; micro-; heavy chain class corresponding to IgM
m	mass; meter; milli-; minim; molar
M	mega-, meg-; molar; moles (per liter); morgan; myopic; myopia
m	moles (per liter)
ⓜ	murmur
$\mu\mu$	micromicro-
μl, μL	microliter
μm	micrometer
mμ	millimicron
mA	milliampere
MA	mental age
MAC *(mak)*	monitored anesthesia care

Abbreviation/ Acronym	Meaning
MAP	morning-after pill
mA-S	milliampere-second
Mb	myoglobin
MBC	maximum breathing capacity
MCP	metacarpophalangeal
MCV	mean corpuscular (cell) volume
MD	muscular dystrophy
MDI	metered-dose inhaler
MEDLARS	Medical Literature Analysis and Retrieval System
MEP	maximal expiratory pressure
meq, mEq	milliequivalent
MET	metabolic equivalent of task
MEV	million electron-volts (10 ev)
mg	milligram
Mg	magnesium
MHA	microhemagglutination
MHC	major histocompatibility complex
MHz	megahertz
MI	myocardial infarction
MICU *(mik′yū)*	medical intensive care unit
MID	minimal infecting dose
MIP	maximum inspiratory pressure
MIS *(mis)*	minimally invasive surgery
MJD	Machado-Joseph disease
ml, mL	milliliter
MLD	minimal lethal dose
mm	millimeter
mm^3, cu mm	cubic millimeter
mmol	millimole
MMPI	Minnesota Multiphasic Personality Inventory

Abbreviation/ Acronym	Meaning
MMR	measles-mumps-rubella (vaccine)
Mn	manganese
MO	medical officer; mineral oil
MODS *(mods)*	multiple organ dysfunction syndrome
mol	mole
mol wt	molecular weight
MOM	milk of magnesia
mono	infectious mononucleosis
MOPP	Mustargen (mechlorethamine hydrochloride), Oncovin (vincristine sulfate), procarbazine hydrochloride, and prednisone
mor. sol.	[L.] *more solito*, as usual, as customary
MPD	maximal permissible dose
MRA	magnetic resonance angiography
mrd, MRD	minimal reacting dose
MRI	magnetic resonance imaging
mRNA	messenger RNA
MRSA	methicillin-resistant *Staphylococcus aureus*
ms, msec	millisecond
MS	multiple sclerosis; morphine sulfate; musculoskeletal
MSG	monosodium glutamate
MSH	melanocyte-stimulating hormone
MTP	metatarsophalangeal (joint)
MUGA *(myū'ga)*	multiple-gated acquisition (imaging)
mV	millivolt
MVP	mitral valve prolapse
MVV	maximal voluntary ventilation
MW	molecular weight
My	myopia

Abbreviation/ Acronym	Meaning
N	newton; nitrogen; normal concentration
N	normal
Na	[Modern L.] *natrium*, sodium
NA	*Nomina Anatomica*
NAD	nicotinamide adenine dinucleotide; no acute distress
NCV	nerve conduction velocity
Ne	neon
NE	norepinephrine; not examined
NEEP	negative end-expiratory pressure
NF	National Formulary
ng	nanogram
NG	nasogastric
Ni	nickel
NICU *(nik'yū)*	neonatal intensive care unit
NK	natural killer (cell)
NKA	no known allergies
NKDA	no known drug allergy
nm	nanometer
noc.	night
NPO	nothing by mouth
NREM	nonrapid eye movement (sleep)
nRNA	nuclear RNA
NS	normal saline
NSAID *(en'sed)*	nonsteroidal anti-inflammatory drug
NSR	normal sinus rhythm
Ω	omega; ohm
o-	ortho-
O	[L.] *oculus*, eye; opening (in formulas for electrical reactions); oxygen; objective
O_2	oxygen
OA	osteoarthritis

Abbreviation/ Acronym	Meaning
OB	obstetrics
OB/GYN	obstetrics and gynecology
OBS	organic brain syndrome
OC	oral contraceptive
OCD	obsessive-compulsive disorder
OCP	oral contraceptive pill
OD	[L.] *oculus dexter*, right eye; overdose
OH	occupational history
OMS	organic mental syndrome
OP	osmotic pressure; outpatient
O&P	ova and parasites
OPV	oral poliovirus vaccine
OR	operating room
ORIF	open reduction, internal fixation
OS	[L.] *oculus sinister*, left eye
OT	occupational therapy; Koch old tuberculin
OTC	over the counter (nonprescription drug)
OU	[L.] *oculus uterque*, each eye (both eyes)
OXT	oxytocin
oz	ounce
$\bar{p}$	after
p	pico-; pupil
p-	para-
P	partial pressure; peta-; phosphorus, phosphoric residue; plasma concentration; pressure; para (obstetric history); plan; posterior; pulse; blood group (PI antigen)
p24	HIV antibody
PA	posterior-anterior
$PaCO_2$	partial pressure of carbon dioxide

Abbreviation/ Acronym	Meaning
PACS *(paks)*	picture archival communications system
PACU *(pak'yū)*	postanesthetic care unit
PALS *(pals)*	pediatric advanced life support
PaO_2	partial pressure of arterial oxygen
Pap	Papanicolaou (smear)
PAR	postanesthetic recovery
Pb	[L.] *plumbum*, lead
p.c.	[L.] *post cibum*, after a meal
Pco_2	partial pressure of carbon dioxide
PD	prism diopter; panic disorder
PDA	patent ductus arteriosus
PDLL	poorly differentiated lymphocytic lymphoma
PE	physical examination; pulmonary embolism; polyethylene
PEEP *(pēp)*	positive end-expiratory pressure
PEFR	peak expiratory flow rate
PEG *(peg)*	percutaneous endoscopic gastrostomy
per	by or through
PERRLA *(pĕr'lă)*	pupils equal, round, and reactive to light and accommodation
PET *(pet)*	positron-emission tomography
PF	peak flow
PFT	pulmonary function test
PG	prostaglandin
pH	hydrogen ion concentration; p (power) of $[H^+]_{10;}$ potential of hydrogen
PH	past history
PI	present illness
PICC	peripherally inserted central catheter
PICU *(pik'yū)*	pediatric intensive care unit
PID	pelvic inflammatory disease

Abbreviation/ Acronym	Meaning
PIH	pregnancy-induced hypertension
PIP *(pip)*	proximal interphalangeal (joint)
PKU	phenylketonuria
PLT	platelet
p.m.	after noon
PM	postmortem
PMH	past medical history
PMN	polymorphonuclear (leukocyte)
PMS	premenstrual syndrome
PND	paroxysmal nocturnal dyspnea; postnasal drip
PNPB	positive-negative pressure breathing
PNS	peripheral nervous system
p.o., PO	[L.] *per os*, by mouth
PO_2, Po_2	partial pressure of oxygen
POMP	prednisone, Oncovin (vincristine sulfate), methotrexate, and Purinethol (6-mercaptopurine)
POR	problem-oriented medical record
post-op, postop	postoperative
PPBS	postprandial blood sugar
ppm	parts per million
PPPPPP	pain, pallor, pulselessness, paresthesia, paralysis, prostration
PPV	positive pressure ventilation
PR	per rectum; progesterone receptor
pre-op, preop	preoperative
p.r.n., PRN	[L.] *pro re nata*, as needed
pro time	prothrombin time
PSA	prostate-specific antigen
PSG	polysomnography
psi	pounds per square inch

Abbreviation/ Acronym	Meaning
PSV	pressure-supported ventilation
pt	patient
PT	physical therapy; prothrombin time
PTA	plasma thromboplastin antecedent; phosphotungstic acid; prior to admission
PTCA	percutaneous transluminal coronary angioplasty
PTH	parathyroid hormone
PT-INR	prothrombin time internal normalized ratio
PTP	posttransfusion purpura
PTSD	posttraumatic stress disorder
PTT	partial thromboplastin time
Pu	plutonium
PUD	peptic ulcer disease
PUO	pyrexia of unknown origin
PUVA (pū ′vă)	psoralen ultraviolet A
PV	per vagina
Px	physical examination
q	every
Q	volume of blood flow
q.d.	[L.] *quaque die*, every day
qh	every hour
q2h	every 2 hours
q.i.d.	[L.] *quater in die*, four times a day
QNS	quantity not sufficient
Qo$_2$	oxygen consumption
q.s.	[L.] *quantum satis*, as much as is enough; [L.] *quantum sufficiat*, as much as may suffice; quantity sufficient
qt	quart
r	racemic; roentgen

Abbreviation/Acronym	Meaning
R	gas constant (8.315 joules); organic radical; Réamur (scale) ; [L.] *recipe*, take; resistance determinant (plasmid); resistance (electrical); resistance (unit; in the cardiovascular system); resolution; respiration; respiratory (exchange ratio); roentgen
®	right
Ra	radium
RA	rheumatoid arthritis
RAI	radioactive iodine
rbc, RBC	red blood cell; red blood (cell) count
RBF	renal blood flow
RD	reaction of degeneration; reaction of denervation
RDA	recommended daily allowance
rDNA	ribosomal DNA
RDS	respiratory distress syndrome
REM *(rem)*	rapid eye movement (sleep); reticular erythematous mucinosis
RF	release factor; rheumatoid factor
RFA	right frontoanterior (fetal position)
RFP	right frontoposterior (fetal position)
RFT	right frontotransverse (fetal position)
Rh	Rhesus (Rh blood group); rhodium
RH	releasing hormone
RhD	rhesus antigen D typing
RLL	right lower lobe
RLQ	right lower quadrant
RMA	right mentoanterior (fetal position)
RML	right middle lobe
RMP	right mentoposterior (fetal position)

Abbreviation/ Acronym	Meaning
RMT	right mentotransverse (fetal position)
Rn	radon
RNA	ribonucleic acid
RNase	ribonuclease
RNP	ribonucleoprotein
R/O	rule out
ROA	right occipitoanterior (fetal position)
ROM	range of motion
ROP	right occipitoposterior (fetal position)
ROS	review of symptoms
ROT	right occipitotransverse (fetal position)
rpm	revolutions per minute
rRNA	ribosomal RNA
RRR	regular rate and rhythm
Rs	resolution
RSA	right sacroanterior (fetal position)
RSP	right sacroposterior (fetal position)
RST	right sacrotransverse (fetal position)
RTC	return to clinic
RTO	return to office
RUL	right upper lobe
RUQ	right upper quadrant
RV	residual volume
RVH	right ventricular hypertrophy
Rx	[L.] *recipe* (the first word on a prescription), take; prescription; treatment
Σ	sigma; reflection coefficient; standard deviation; 1 millisecond (0.001 sec)
s	[L.] *semis*, half; steady state (subscript); [L.] *sinister*, left

Abbreviation/ Acronym	Meaning
S	[L.] *sinister*, left; saturation of hemoglobin (percentage of; followed by subscript O_2 or CO_2); siemens; spherical; spherical lens; sulfur; Svedberg unit; subjective
$\bar{s}$	without
SA, S-A	sinoatrial
SAB	spontaneous abortion
SAD *(sad)*	seasonal affective disorder
SaO_2	oxygen saturation of arterial (oxyhemoglobin)
SARS *(sarz)*	severe acute respiratory syndrome
sat.	saturated
sat. sol.	saturated solution
sc	subcutaneous(ly)
SC	sternoclavicular; subcutaneous(ly)
SCC	squamous cell carcinoma
Se	selenium
SERM *(serm)*	selective estrogen receptor modulator
SGOT	serum glutamic-oxaloacetic transaminase (aspartate aminotransferase)
SGPT	serum glutamic-pyruvic transaminase (alanine aminotransferase)
SH	serum hepatitis; social history
Si	silicon
SIDS *(sids)*	sudden infant death syndrome
sig.	[L.] *signa*, affix a label, inscribe
SIMV	spontaneous intermittent mandatory ventilation; synchronized intermittent mandatory ventilation

Abbreviation/ Acronym	Meaning
SIRS *(sěrs)*	systemic inflammatory response syndrome
SK	streptokinase
SLE	systemic lupus erythematosus
SLR	straight leg raising
SMAC *(smak)*	sequential multiple analyzer computer
Sn	[L.] *stannum*, tin
SOAP *(sep)*	subjective data, objective data, assessment, and plan (problem-oriented medical record)
SOB	short(ness) of breath
sol., soln.	solution
sp.	species
SPECT *(spek)*	single-photon emission computed tomography
SPF	sun protection factor
sp. gr., SpGr	specific gravity
spm	suppression and mutation
spp.	species (plural)
SQ	subcutaneous
Sr	strontium
SR	systems review
ssDNA	single-stranded DNA
ssp.	subspecies
ST	scapulothoracic
stat, STAT	[L.] *statim*, immediately, at once
STD	sexually transmitted disease
STM	short-term memory
SUI	stress urinary incontinence
suppos	suppository
SV	stroke volume
SVT	supraventricular tachycardia

Abbreviation/ Acronym	Meaning
Sx	symptom
t	metric ton
t	temperature (Celsius); tritium
T	temperature absolute (Kelvin)
T	temperature; tension (intraocular); tera-; tesla; tetanus (toxoid); tidal (volume) (subscript); tocopherol; transverse (tubule); tritium; tumor (antigen)
T_3, T3	3,5,5′-triiodothyronine
T_4, T4	tetraiodothyronine (thyroxine)
TA	*Terminologia Anatomica*
T&A	tonsillectomy and adenoidectomy
tab	tablet
TAB	therapeutic abortion
TAF	tumor angiogenesis factor
TB	tuberculosis
Tc	technetium
^{99m}Tc	technetium-99m
T&C	type and crossmatch
TCN	talocalcaneonavicular (joint)
Td	tetanus-diphtheria (toxoids, adult type)
TEDS	thromboembolic disease stockings
TEE	transesophageal echocardiogram
TENS *(tens)*	transcutaneous electrical nerve stimulation
Ti	titanium
TIA	transient ischemic attack
TIBC	total iron-binding capacity
t.i.d.	[L.] *ter in die*, three times a day
tinct.	tincture
TKO	to keep (venous infusion line) open

Abbreviation/ Acronym	Meaning
Tl	thallium
TLC	thin-layer chromatography; total lung capacity; tender loving care
TLV	threshold-limit value
TM	transport maximum; tympanic membrane
TMJ	temporomandibular joint
TMT	tarsometatarsal
TNF	tumor necrosis factor
TNM	tumor, node, metastasis (tumor staging)
t-PA, tPA, TPA	tissue plasminogen activator
TPN	total parenteral nutrition
TPR	temperature, pulse, and respirations
tr.	tincture
Tr	treatment
tRNA	transfer RNA
TRUS *(trŭs)*	transrectal ultrasound
TSH	thyroid-stimulating hormone
TSS	toxic shock syndrome
TTP	thrombotic thrombocytopenic purpura
TU	toxic unit, toxin unit
TURP *(tŭrp)*	transurethral resection of the prostate
TV	tidal volume
Tx	treatment; traction
U	unit; uranium; uridine (in polymers); urinary (concentration)
UA	urinalysis
UCHD	usual childhood diseases
UGIS	upper gastrointestinal series
ung.	[L.] *unguentum*, ointment
u-PA	urokinase
URI	upper respiratory infection

Abbreviation/Acronym	Meaning
US, U/S	ultrasound
UTI	urinary tract infection
UV	ultraviolet
v	venous (blood); volt
V	vanadium; vision; visual (acuity); volt; volume (frequently with subscripts denoting location, chemical species, and conditions)
$\dot{V}$	ventilation; gas flow (frequently with subscripts indicating location and chemical species); ventilation
VA	viral antigen
V-A	ventriculoatrial
VATS (vats)	video-assisted thoracic surgery
VC	vision, color; vital capacity
VCE	vagina, (ecto)cervix, endocervical canal
VCU, VCUG	voiding cystourethrogram
V_D	(physiologic) dead space
VDRL	Venereal Disease Research Laboratory (test)
VHDL	very-high-density lipoprotein
VLDL	very-low-density lipoprotein
V_{max}	maximal velocity
VP	vasopressin; Voges-Proskauer
V/Q	ventilation/perfusion
VS	volumetric solution; vital signs
VSD	ventricular septal defect
V_T	tidal volume
w.a.	while awake
W	watt; [German] Wolfram, tungsten
WBC	white blood cell; white blood (cell) count
WD	well developed

Abbreviation/ Acronym	Meaning
WDLL	well-differentiated lymphocytic (or lymphatic) lymphoma
WDWN	well developed, well nourished
wk	week
WN	well nourished
WNL	within normal limits
WNV	West Nile virus
Wt	weight
x	times; for
x-ray	radiography
y.o., y/o	year old
yr	year

Symbols

Symbol	Meaning
Angles, Triangles, and Circles	
$\wedge$	above; diastolic blood pressure (anesthesia records); elevated; enlarged; improved; increased; superior (position); upper
$\vee$	below; decreased; deficiency; deficit; depressed; deteriorated; diminished; down; inferior (position); lower; systolic blood pressure (anesthesia records)
$>$	causes; demonstrates; distal; followed by; derived from; greater than*; indicates; leads to; more severe than; produces; radiates to; radiating to; results in reveals; shows; to; toward; worse than; yields
$<$	caused by; derived from; less severe than; less than*; produced by; proximal
$\angle$	angle; flexion; flexor
$\angle\!\!\!\!/E$	angle of entry
$\angle\!\!\!\!/x$	angle of exit
$\llcorner$	factorial product
$\lrcorner$	right lower quadrant
$\urcorner$	right upper quadrant
$\ulcorner$	left upper quadrant
$\llcorner$	left lower quadrant
Δ	anion gap; centrad prism; change; delta gap; heat; increment; occipital triangle; prism diopter; temperature (anesthesia records)
$\Delta+$	time interval
$\Delta\,A$	change in absorbance
Δ dB	difference in decibels

*Do not use in written patient records (JCAHO).

Symbol	Meaning
Δ P	change in (intraocular) pressure
Δ pH	change in pH
Δ t	time interval
Δ H, HΔ	Hesselbach triangle
○	respiration (anesthesia records)
♀	female, female sex
♂	male, male sex
Ⓐ, ⓐx	axilla (temperature)
Ⓗ, ⓗ	hypodermic(ally)
ⒾⓂ	intramuscular(ly)
ⒾⓋ	intravenous intravenously
Ⓛ	left
Ⓜ	murmur
ⓜ	by mouth; mouth (temperature); murmur
√ⓜ	factitial murmur
Ⓞ	by mouth; oral; orally
Ⓡ	rectal; rectally; rectum (temperature); right
Ⓧ	end of anesthesia (anesthesia records); end of operation

Arrows

↑	above; elevated; elevation; enlarged; gas; greater than; improved; increase; increased; increases; more than; rising; superior (position); up; upper
↑ g	increasing; rising
↑ V	increase due to in vivo effect (laboratory)

Symbol	Meaning
↓	below; decrease; decreased; deficiency; deficit; depressed; depression; deteriorated; deteriorating; diminished; diminution; down; falling; inferior (position); less than; low; normal plantar reflex; precipitate; precipitates; slower
↓ g	decreasing; diminishing; falling; lowering
↓ V	decrease due to in vivo effect (laboratory)
↗	deviated; displaced; increasing
↘	decreasing
→	approaches; limit of; causes, demonstrates; direction of flow or reaction; distal; due to; followed by; indicates; leads to; produces; radiating to; results in; reveals; shows to; to; right; toward; yields
←	caused by; derived from; direction of flow or reaction; due to; produced by; proximal; resulting from; secondary to; to left
↑↑	extensor response (up bilaterally, positive Babinski sign); testes undescended
↓↓	plantar response (down bilaterally, normal Babinski sign); testes descended
↓↑	reversible reaction; up and down
⇄, ⇌	reversible (chemical) reaction

Symbol	Meaning

Genetic Symbols

Symbol	Meaning
□	male
○	female
◇	sex unspecified
□ ○	normal individuals
■●◆	affected individual (with ≥ 2 conditions, the symbol is partitioned and shaded with a different fill defined in a key or legend)
⑤⑥⑤	multiple individuals, number known (number of siblings written inside symbol)
ⓝⓝ⟐	multiple individuals, number unknown ("n" used in place of specific number)
□─○	mating
□═○	consanguinity
(+)	uncommon or uncertain mode of inheritance
I □─○ II ○ □	parents and offspring, in generations
⌒○	dizygotic twins
⌒○	monozygotic twins
④ ③	number of children of sex indicated 4
[□] [○]	adopted individuals
⚲ ♀	individual died without leaving offspring
□┬○	no issue
■ ●	affected individuals
↗■ ↗●	proband or propositus (first affected family member coming to medical attention)
⊞	examined professionally normal for trait
⊞	not examined dubiously reported to have trait
□	not examined reliably reported to have trait
◧ ◖	heterozygotes for autosomal recessive
⊙	carrier of sex-linked recessive
⌀⌀	death

Symbol	Meaning
◩ ⊘ ⊗ SB SB SB 28 wk 30 wk 34 wk	stillbirth (SB)
▨ Ⓟ ⟡ LMP: 20 wk 7/1/94	pregnancy (P); gestational age and karotype (if known) below symbol
⟋▢ ⟋○	consultand (individual seeking genetic counseling/testing)
△ △ △ male female ECT	spontaneous abortion (SAB); ECT below symbol indicates ectopic pregnancy
▲ ▲ ▲ male female 16 wk	affected spontaneous abortion (gestational age, if known, below symbol, and key or legend used to define shading)
⧄ ⧄ ⧄ male female	termination of pregnancy
◮ ◮ ◮ male female	affected termination of pregnancy (key or legend used to define shading)

Numbers

0	completely absent (pulse); no response (reflexes)
+1, 1+	markedly impaired (pulse)
1+	low normal or somewhat diminished (reflexes); slight reaction or trace (laboratory tests)
+2, 2+	moderately impaired (pulse)
2+	average or normal (reflexes); noticeable reaction or trace (laboratory tests)
+3, 3+	slightly impaired (pulse)
3+	moderate reaction (laboratory tests); brisker than average (reflexes)
+4, 4+	normal (pulse)
4+	hyperactive (reflexes); large amount (laboratory tests); pronounced reaction (laboratory tests)
•	very brisk (reflexes)
$\overline{1}$	bowel movement (numeral indicates number of stools in a given period)
1×	once; one time
2×, ×2	twice; two times
3×, ×3	three times, etc.

Symbol	Meaning
Arabic	Roman
0	
1	I, i
2	II, ii
3	III, iii
4	IV, iv
5	V, v
6	VI, vi
7	VII, vii
8	VIII, viii
9	IX, ix
10	X, x
11	XI, xi
12	XII, xii
13	XIII, xiii
14	XIV, xiv
15	XV
16	XVI
17	XVII
18	XVIII
19	XIX
20	XX
30	XXX
40	XL
50	L
60	LX
70	LXX
80	LXXX
90	XC
100	C
1,000	M
5,000	$\overline{V}$
10,000	$\overline{X}$

Symbol	Meaning
100,000	$\overline{\text{C}}$
1,000,000	$\overline{\text{M}}$

Pluses, Minuses, and Equivalencies

+	acid (reaction); added to*; convex lens; decreased or diminished (reflexes); excess less than 50% inhibition of hemolysis, Wassermann; low normal (reflexes); markedly impaired (pulse); mild (severity); plus*; positive (laboratory tests); present slight reaction or trace (laboratory tests); sluggish (reflexes); somewhat diminished (reflexes)
(+)	significant
(+)ive	positive
+ to ++	slight pain
++	average (reflexes); 50% inhibition of hemolysis, Wassermann; moderate (pain, severity); moderately impaired (pulse); normally active (reflexes); noticeable reaction or trace (laboratory tests)
+++	increased reflexes; 75% inhibition of hemolysis, Wassermann; moderate amount; moderate reaction (laboratory tests); moderately hyperative (reflexes); moderately severe (pain, severity); brisker than average (reflexes); slightly impaired (pulse)
++++	complete inhibition of hemolysis, Wassermann; large amount (laboratory tests); markedly hyperactive (reflexes); markedly severe (pain, severity); normal (pulse); pronounced reaction (laboratory tests); very brisk (reflexes)
−	absent; alkaline (reaction); concave lens; deficiency; deficient; minus; negative (laboratory test); none; subtract; without
(−)	insignificant

Symbol	Meaning
±	doubtful; either positive or; negative; equivocal (reflexes, qualitative tests); flicker (reflexes); indefinite; more or less; plus or minus; possibly significant; questionable; suggestive; variable very slight (reaction, severity, trace); with or without
(±)	possibly significant
± to ±	minimal pain
∓	minus or plus
‡	moderate (severity); normally active (reflexes)
#	fracture; gauge; number; pound(s); weight
~	about; approximate; approximately; proportionate to
≈	approximately equal to
=	equal to
≠	not equal to
◠	combined with
⇔	equivalent
⇎	not equivalent to
≡	identical; identical with
≢	not identical; not identical with
≑	nearly equal to
≐	approximately equal
≅	approximately; approximately equal to; congruent to
≐	approaches
=	equilateral
△	equiangular
>	greater than*
≯	not greater than
<	less than*
≮	not less than
≥	greater than or equal to
≤	less than or equal to

*Do not use in written patient records (JCAHO).

Symbol	Meaning

Primes, Checks, Dots, Roots, and Other Symbols

Symbol	Meaning
?	doubtful; equivocal (reflexes); flicker (reflexes); not tested (severity); possible; questionable; question of; suggested; suggestive (severity); unknown
!	factorial product
†	death; deceased
/	divided by; either meaning; extension; extensors fraction; of; per*; to; ratio
'	foot; hour; univalent
"	bivalent; ditto; inch; minute; second (1/60 degree)
'''	line ($\sqrt{12}$ inch); trivalent
$\sqrt{}$	check; observe for; urine; voided (urine)
$\sqrt{\cdot}$	urine and defecation; voided and bowels moved
$\sqrt{c}$	check with
$\sqrt{d}$	checked; observed
$\sqrt{g}$, $\sqrt{ing}$	checking
$\sqrt{qs}$	voided quantity sufficient
$\sqrt{}$	radical root
$\sqrt[2]{}$	square root
$\sqrt[3]{}$	cube root
*	birth multiplication sign (genetics); not verified; presumed; supposed
°	degree, measurement (1/360 of circle); severity (burns, wounds); temperature; time (hour)*
:	is to
...	no data (in given category)
∴	therefore
∵	because; since
::	as; equality between ratios; proportion; proportionate to

*Do not use in written patient records (JCAHO).

Symbol	Meaning
Statistical Symbols	
α	probability of Type I error; significance level
β	probability of Type II error
$1-\beta$	power of statistical test
	binomial coefficient
$n^c k; (n/k)$	number of combination of n things taken k at a time
χ^2	chi-squared statistic
E	expected frequency in cell of contingency table
$E(X)$	expected value of random variable X
F	F statistic (variance ratio)
f	frequency
H_0	null hypothesis
H_1	alternative hypothesis
μ	population mean
N	population size
n	sample size
$n!$	n factorial
O	observed frequency in a contingency table
φ	ability continuum phi coefficient
P	probability
p	probability of success in independent trials
$P(A)$	probability that event A occurs
$P(A\backslash B)$	conditional probability that A occurs given that B has occurred
r	sample correlation coefficient, usually the Pearson product-moment correlation
r^2	coefficient of determination
r_s	Spearman rank correlation coefficient
ρ	population correlation coefficient
s	sample standard deviation
s^2	sample variance

Symbol	Meaning
SE	standard error of estimate
σ	population standard deviation
σ^2	population variance
σdiff.	standard error of difference between scores
σest.	standard error of estimate
σmeas.	standard error of measurement
t	Student t statistic; Student test variable
θ	latent trait
U	Mann-Whitney rank sum statistic
W	Wilcoxon rank sum statistic
$\overline{X}$	sample mean
$|x|$	absolute value of x
$\sqrt{x}$	square root of x
Z	standard score
∞	infinity

Dangerous Abbreviations

The Joint Commission on Accreditation of Healthcare Organizations (JCAHO; www.jcaho.org) published a list of dangerous abbreviations, acronyms, and symbols not to be used. It was originally created in 2004 and updated in May 2005.

As of May 2005, the survey and scoring of this requirement applies to all orders and all medication-related documentation that is handwritten (including free-text computer entry) or on preprinted forms.

JCAHO "Do Not Use" List

Abbreviation	Potential Problem	Preferred Term
U (for unit)	Mistaken as 0 (zero), 4 (four), or cc	Write "unit"
IU (for international unit)	Mistaken as IV (intravenous) or 10 (ten)	Write "international unit"
Q.D., QD, q.d., qd (daily)	Mistaken for each other	Write "daily"
Q.O.D., QOD, q.o.d, qod (every other day)	Period after the "Q" mistaken for "I" and the "O" mistaken for "I"	Write "every other day"
Trailing zero (X.0 mg), lack of leading zero (.X mg)	Decimal point is missed.	Never write a zero by itself after a decimal point (X mg)* Always use a zero before a decimal point (0.X mg)
MS, MSO_4, and $MgSO_4$	Can mean morphine sulfate or magnesium sulfate	Write "morphine sulfate"
	Confused for one another	Write "magnesium sulfate"

*Exception: a "trailing zero" may be used only where required to demonstrate the level of precision of the value being reported, such as for laboratory results, imaging studies that report size of lesions, or catheter/tube sizes. It may not be used in medication orders or other medication-related documentation.

An abbreviation on the do-not-use list should not be used in any forms—upper or lower case, with or without periods. For example, if Q.D. is on your list, you cannot use QD or qd. Any of those variations may be confusing and could be misinterpreted.

Additional Abbreviations, Acronyms, and Symbols That Should Be Avoided

Abbreviation	Potential problem	Preferred term
> (greater than), < (less than)	Mistaken for 7 (seven) or the letter "L"; confused for one another	Write "greater than" or "less than"
Abbreviations for drug names	Misinterpreted due to similar abbreviations for multiple drugs	Write drug names in full
Apothecary units	Unfamiliar to many practitioners; confused with metric units	Use metric units
@	Mistaken for 2 (two)	Write "at"
cc (for cubic centimeter)	Mistaken for U (units) when poorly written	Write "ml" or "milliliters"
μg (for microgram)	Mistaken for mg (milligrams), resulting in one thousand-fold overdose	Write "mcg" or "micrograms"

Healthcare Organizations

Abbreviation	Organization
AABB	American Association of Blood Banks
AACAP	American Academy of Child and Adolescent Psychiatry
AACC	American Association for Clinical Chemistry
AACD	American Academy of Cosmetic Dentistry
AACN	American Association of Critical-Care Nurses
AACOM	American Association of Colleges of Osteopathic Medicine
AACR	American Association for Cancer Research
AACVPR	American Association of Cardiovascular and Pulmonary Rehabilitation
AAD	American Academy of Dermatology
AAE	American Association of Endodontists
AAFP	American Academy of Family Physicians
AAGP	American Association for Geriatric Psychiatry
AAHP	American Association of Homeopathic Pharmacists
AAI	American Association of Immunologists
AAM	American Academy of Microbiologists
AAMA	American Academy of Medical Acupuncture
AAMD	American Association on Mental Deficiency
AAMFT	American Association for Marriage and Family Therapists
AAMI	Association for the Advancement of Medical Instrumentation
AAMR	American Association on Mental Retardation
AAN	American Academy of Neurology; American Association of Neuropathologists
AANA	American Association of Nurse Anesthetists
AANP	American Association of Naturopathic Physicians

Abbreviation	Organization
AAO	American Academy of Ophthalmology
AAOA	American Academy of Otolaryngic Allergy
AAO-HNS	American Academy of Otolaryngology-Head and Neck Surgery
AAOS	American Academy of Orthopaedic Surgeons
AAP	American Academy of Pediatrics; American Association of Pathologists
AAPB	American Association of Pathologists and Bacteriologists; Association for Applied Psychophysiology and Biofeedback
AAPCC	American Association of Poison Control Centers
AAPMR	American Academy of Physical Medicine and Rehabilitation
AARP	American Association of Retired Persons
AASLD	American Association for the Study of Liver Diseases
AAST	American Association for the Surgery of Trauma
AAWC	American Academy of Wound Management
ABA	American Bar Association; American Board of Anesthesiology
ABC	American Botanical Council
ABIM	American Board of Internal Medicine
ABMTR	Autologous Bone Marrow Transplant Registry
ABPH	American Board of Psychological Hypnosis
ABPN	American Board of Psychiatry and Neurology
ABR	American Board of Radiology
ABS	American Board of Surgery
ABTA	American Brain Tumor Association
ACA	American Chiropractic Association; American Counseling Association
ACB	American Council of the Blind
ACC	American College of Cardiology

Abbreviation	Organization
ACC/AHA	American College of Cardiology/American Heart Association
ACG	American College of Gastroenterology
ACIP	Advisory Committee on Immunization Practices
ACLA	American Clinical Laboratory Association
ACLPS	Academy of Clinical Laboratory Physicians and Scientists
ACNM	American College of Nurse-Midwives
ACNP	American College of Nurse Practitioners
ACOG	American College of Obstetricians and Gynecologists
ACP	American College of Pathologists
ACP-ASIM	American College of Physicians-American Society of Internal Medicine
ACR	American College of Radiology; American College of Rheumatology
ACS	American Cancer Society; American Chemical Society; American College of Surgeons; Association of Clinical Scientists
ACSM	American College of Sports Medicine
ADA	American Dental Association; American Diabetes Association; American Dietetic Association
ADHF	American Digestive Health Foundation
AEC	American Endosonography Club; Atomic Energy Commission
AFS	American Fertility Society
AGA	American Gastroenterological Association
AGD	Academy of General Dentistry
AHA	American Heart Association; American Hospital Association

Abbreviation	Organization
AHDI	Association for Healthcare Documentation Integrity
AHFS-DI	American Hospital Formulary Service-Drug Information
AHHA	American Holistic Health Association
AHIMA	American Health Information Management Association
AHTA	American Horticultural Therapy Association
AIN	American Institute of Nutrition
AIP	American Institute of Physics
AIUM	American Institute of Ultrasound in Medicine
AJCC	American Joint Committee on Cancer
AJCC/UICC	American Joint Committee on Cancer/International Union Against Cancer
AMA	American Medical Association
AMA-DE	American Medical Association Drug Evaluation
AMDA	American Medical Directors Association
AME	American Medical Electronics
AMF	American Menopause Foundation
AMPAC	Alternative Medicine Program Advisory Council
AMT	American Medical Technologists
AMTA	American Massage Therapy Association; American Music Therapy Association
ANA	American Nurses Association
ANRC	American National Red Cross
AOA	American Optometric Association; American Orthopaedic Association; American Osteopathic Association
AOFAS	American Orthopaedic Foot and Ankle Society
AORN	Association of Perioperative Registered Nurses
AOTA	American Occupational Therapy Association, Inc.

Abbreviation	Organization
APA	American Psychiatric Association; American Psychological Association
APMA	American Podiatric Medical Association
APNA	American Psychiatric Nurses Association
APSA	American Pediatric Surgical Association
APTA	American Physical Therapy Association
ARA	American Rheumatism Association
ARC	American Red Cross; Association for Retarded Citizens
ARCBS	American Red Cross Blood Services
ARDMS	American Registry of Diagnostic Medical Sonographers
ARN	Association of Rehabilitation Nurses
ASA	American Society of Anesthesiologists; American Society on Aging; American Standards Association; American Stroke Association
ASAPS	American Society for Aesthetic Plastic Surgery
ASB	American Society of Bacteriologists
ASCCP	American Society for Colposcopy and Cervical Pathology
ASCI	American Society for Clinical Investigation
ASCIA	American Spinal Cord Injury Association
ASCLT	American Society of Clinical Laboratory Technicians
ASCP	American Society of Clinical Pathologists
ASCRS	American Society for Colon and Rectal Surgeons
ASEP	American Society for Experimental Pathology
ASGE	American Society for Gastrointestinal Endoscopy
ASH	American Society of Hematology

Abbreviation	Organization
ASHA	American Speech-Language-Hearing Association
ASIA	American Spinal Injury Association
ASIF	Association for the Study of Internal Fixation
ASIM	American Society of Internal Medicine
ASM	American Society for Microbiologists
ASP	American Society of Pathologists
ASPO	American Society of Preventive Oncology
ASPRS	American Society of Plastic and Reconstructive Surgeons
ASPS	American Society of Plastic Surgeons
ASRT	American Society of Radiologic Technologists
ASSH	American Society for Surgery of the Hand
ASTM	American Society for Testing and Materials
ASTRO	American Society for Therapeutic Radiology and Oncology
ASTS	American Society of Transplant Surgeons
ATA	American Tinnitus Association
ATPO	Association of Technical Personnel in Ophthalmology
ATS	American Thoracic Society
AUA	American Urological Association
AUR	Association of University Radiologists
BDAC	Bureau of Drug Abuse Control
BHP	Bureau of Health Professions
BNIST	National Bureau of Scientific Information
CAFMHS	Child, Adolescent, and Family Mental Health Service
CAP	College of American Pathologists
CCNSC	Cancer Chemotherapy National Service Center
CDB	Center for Drugs and Biologics
CDC, CDCP	Centers for Disease Control and Prevention

Abbreviation	Organization
CDHNF	Children's Digestive Health and Nutrition Foundation
CDRH	Center for Devices and Radiological Health
CEM	Center for Molecular Epidemiology
CFH	Council on Family Health
CHAS	Center for Health Administration Studies
CHC	Community Health Council
CIP	Carcinogen Information Program; Cardiac Injury Panel
CLMA	Clinical Laboratory Management Association
CMB	Central Midwives' Board
CMHS	Center for Mental Health Services
CNME	Council on Naturopathic Medical Education
CODATA	Committee on Data for Science and Technology
COLA	Commission on Office Laboratory Accreditation
COTH	Council of Teaching Hospitals
CPEHS	Consumer Protection and Environmental Health Service
CPHA	Commission on Professional and Hospital Activities
CPSC	Consumer Product Safety Commission
CREOG	Council on Resident Education in Obstetrics and Gynecology
CRHL	Collaborative Radiological Health Laboratory
CRRMP	Committee of Radiation from Radioactive Medicinal Products
CSIN	Chemical Substances Information Network
CSM	Committee on Safety of Medicines
CSMB	Center for Study of Multiple Births
CSTI	Clearinghouse for Scientific and Technical Information
CSU	Central Statistical Unit (of Venereal Disease Research Laboratory)

Abbreviation	Organization
CTDTADA	The Council on Dental Therapeutics of the American Dental Association
DAC	Division of Ambulatory Care
DAHEA	Department of Allied Health Education and Accreditation
DAWN	Drug Abuse Warning Network
DDNC	Digestive Disease National Coalition
DEBRA	Dystrophic Epidermolysis Bullosa Research Association of America
DEHS	Division of Emergency Health Services
DEM	Department of Emergency Medicine
DGMS	Division of General Medical Services
DHES	Division of Health Examination Statistics
DHHS	Department of Health and Human Services
DHI	Dental Health International
DHS	Department of Human Services
DLC	Dental Laboratory Conference
DMH	Department of Mental Health; Department of Mental Hygiene
DMS	Department of Medicine and Surgery
DOH	Department of Health
DOSS	Department of Social Services
DRME	Division of Research in Medical Education
DSHS	Department of Social and Health Services
DSMB	Data and Safety Monitoring Board
DSS	Department of Social Services
DTBE	Division of Tuberculosis Elimination
DVA	Department of Veterans Affairs
DVCC	Disease Vector Control Center
DVH	Division for the Visually Handicapped
DVR	Division of Vocational Rehabilitation
EAB	Ethics Advisory Board
EBAA	Eye Bank Association of America

Abbreviation	Organization
EC	Enzyme Commission (of International Union of Biochemistry)
ECFMG	Educational Commission on Foreign Medical Graduates
EHA	Environmental Health Administration
EHPAC	Emergency Health Preparedness Advisory Committee
EIS	Epidemic Intelligence Service
ELSO	Extracorporeal Life Support Organization
EMCRO	Experimental Medical Care Review Organization
EPI	Expanded Program of Immunizations (World Health Organization)
FACNHA	Foundation of American College of Nursing Home Administrators
FACOSH	Federal Advisory Council on Occupational Safety and Health
FAH	Federation of American Hospitals
FBR	Foundation for Biomedical Research
FCER	Foundation for Chiropractic Education and Research
FCIC	Federal Consumer Information Center
FCMW	Foundation for Child Mental Welfare
FIGO	International Federation of Gynecology and Obstetrics
FOA	Federation of Orthodontic Associations
FPO	Federation of Prosthodontic Organizations
GDC	General Dental Council
GMENAC	Graduate Medical Education National Advisory Committee
GNC	General Nursing Council
GOG	Gynecologic Oncology Group (of National Cancer Institute)

Abbreviation	Organization
GPA	Global Program on AIDS
GRF	Glaucoma Research Foundation
GSA	Gerontological Society of America
HAP	Handicapped Aid Program
HCA	Hospital Corporation of America
HCFA	Health Care Financing Administration
HCRE	Homeopathic Council for Research and Education
HDRF	Heart Disease Research Foundation
HDSA	Huntington's Disease Society of America
HEC	Health Education Council
HeCOG	Hellenic Cooperative Oncology Group
HER	HIV Epidemiology Research
HERS	Hysterectomy Educational Resources and Services Foundation
HHS	(Department of) Health and Human Services
HIAA	Health Insurance Association of America
HIBAC	Health Insurance Benefits Advisory Council
HIC	Heart Information Center
HICPAC	Hospital Infection Control Practices Advisory Committee
HII	Health Insurance Institute
HIVNET	Human Immunodeficiency Virus Project Network
HMSS	Hospital Management Systems Society
HNCCG	Head and Neck Cancer Cooperative Group
HAS	Health Services Administration
IADR	International Association for Dental Research
IAET	International Association for Enterostomal Therapy
IAG	International Academy of Gnathology
IAO	International Association for Orthodontics
IAP	International Academy of Pathology

Abbreviation	Organization
IAPAAS	International Association of Physical Activity, Aging, and Sports
IAPG	International Antimicrobial Project Group
IARC	International Agency for Research on Cancer
IASHS	Institute for Advanced Study in Human Sexuality
IASP	International Association for the Study of Pain
IAVI	International AIDS Vaccine Initiative
IBC	Institutional Biosafety Committee
IBCSG	International Breast Cancer Study Group
IBMTR	International Bone Marrow Transplant Registry
ICA	Institute of Clinical Analysis; International Chiropractic Association
ICAAC	Interscience Conference on Antimicrobial Agents and Chemotherapy
ICCIDD	International Council for Control of Iodine Deficiency Disorder
ICCR	International Committee for Contraceptive Research
ICDRG	International Contact Dermatitis Research Group
ICHD	Inter-Society Commission for Heart Disease
ICHPPC	International Classification of Health Problems in Primary Care
ICIC	International Cancer Information Center
ICOPER	International Cooperative Pulmonary Embolism Registry
ICR	Institute for Cancer Research
ICRETT	International Cancer Research Technology Transfer
ICREW	International Cancer Research Workshop
ICRP	International Commission on Radiological Protection

Abbreviation	Organization
ICS	International Continence Society
ICSH	International Committee for Standardization in Hematology
IDSA	Infectious Disease Society of America
IEC	Independent Ethics Committee
IFCC	International Federation of Clinical Chemistry
IFRP	International Fertility Research Program
IGCCCG	International Germ Cell Cancer Collaborative Group
IHCP	Institute of Hospital and Community Psychiatry
IHS	Indian Health Service; International Headache Society
IIME	Institute of International Medical Education
IIS	International Institute of Stress
IKDC	International Knee Documentation Committee
ILAE	International League Against Epilepsy
ILAR	International League of Associations for Rheumatology
IMIC	International Medical Information Center
IMR	Institute for Medical Research; Institution for the Mentally Retarded
IMRG	Internal Microvascular Research Group
IOA	International Ostomy Association
IOM	Institute of Medicine
IPAR	Institute of Personality Assessment and Research
IRC	Institutional Review Committee (Board); International Red Cross
IRH	Institute of Religion and Health; Institute for Research in Hypnosis
IRIS	International Research Information Service
IRSG	Intergroup Rhabdomyosarcoma Study Group

Abbreviation	Organization
ISCLT	International Society for Clinical Laboratory Technology
ISCP	International Society of Comparative Pathology
ISGyP	International Society of Gynecologic Pathologists
ISH	International Society of Hematology
ISHLT	International Society for Heart and Lung Transplantation
ISHT	International Society for Heart Transplantation
ISM	International Society of Microbiologists
ISMP	Institute for Safe Medication Practices
ISO	International Standards Organization
ISR	Institute for Sex Research; Institute of Surgical Research
ISSVD	International Society for the Study of Vulvar Diseases
ISUP	International Society for Urological Pathology
ITC	Interagency Testing Committee
ITF	International Tremor Foundation
ITI	International Team Implantologists
ITQB-IBET	Molecular Genetics Unit of the Institute of Biotechnology
IUPAC	International Union of Pure and Applied Chemistry
JCAHO	Joint Commission on Accreditation of Healthcare Organizations
JCAHPO	Joint Commission on Allied Health Personnel in Ophthalmology
JCMHC	Joint Commission on Mental Health of Children
JDF	Juvenile Diabetes Foundation
JRCOMP	Joint Review Committee for Ophthalmic Medical Personnel

Abbreviation	Organization
LCSSG	Laparoscopic Colorectal Surgery Group
MCB	Medicines Control Board
MCR	Medical Corps Reserve
MGMA	Medical Group Management Association
MHA	Mental Health Association
MHCS	Mental Hygiene Consultation Service
MHI	Mental Health Institute
MHRI	Mental Health Research Institute
MLA	Medical Library Association
MMPNC	Medical Maternal Program for Nuclear Casualties
MMRS	Metropolitan Medical Response Systems
MSSP	Maternal Support Services Program
MSTS	Musculoskeletal Tumor Society
MTF	Musculoskeletal Transplant Foundation
MTSO	Medical Transcription Service Organization
N4A	National Association of Area Agencies on Aging
NAACLS	National Accrediting Agency for Clinical Laboratory Sciences
NAAMM	North American Academy of Manipulative Medicine
NACDG	North American Contact Dermatitis Group
NACHC	National Association of Community Health Centers
NACI	National Advisory Committee on Immunization
NACSCAOM	National Accreditation Commission for Schools and Colleges of Acupuncture and Oriental Medicine
NAD	National Association of the Deaf
NADL	National Association of Dental Laboratories
NAEPP	National Asthma Education and Prevention Program
NAFC	National Association for Continence

Abbreviation	Organization
NAHC	National Association for Home Care
NAHD	National Association for Human Development
NAHF	National Association for Health & Fitness
NAHI	National Athletic Health Institute
NAHOF	National Association on HIV Over Fifty
NAMCS	National Ambulatory Medical Care Survey
NAMI	National Alliance for the Mentally Ill
NAMS	North American Menopause Society
NANASP	National Association of Nutrition and Aging Service Programs
NANDA	North American Nursing Diagnosis Association
NAPGCM	National Association of Progressional Geriatric Care Managers
NAPNAP	National Association of Pediatric Nurse Associates and Practitioners
NAPNES	National Association for Practical Nurse Education and Services
NARIC	National Rehabilitation Information Center
NASPGN	North American Society for Pediatric Gastroenterology and Nutrition
NATR	National Association of Tumor Registrars
NBCCG	National Bladder Cancer Collaborative Group
NBTS	National Blood Transfusion Service
NCADD	National Council on Alcoholism and Drug Dependence
NCAHE	National Council Against Health Fraud
NCAI	National Coalition for Adult Immunization
NCAMLP	National Certification Agency for Medical Laboratory Personnel
NCBA	National Caucus and Center on Black Aged, Inc.
NCCAM	National Center for Complementary and Alternative Medicine

Abbreviation	Organization
NCCAN	National Center for Child Abuse and Neglect
NCCAOM	National Certification Committee for Acupuncture and Oriental Medicine
NCCDS	National Cooperative Collaborative Crohn's Disease Study
NCCLS	National Committee for Clinical Laboratory Standards
NCCN	National Comprehensive Cancer Network
NCCNHR	National Citizen's Coalition for Nursing Home Reform
NCCS	National Coalition for Cancer Survivorship
NCCTG	North Central Cancer Treatment Group
NCDB	National Cancer Data Base
NCEA	National Center on Elder Abuse
NCEP	National Cholesterol Education Program
NCHLS	National Council of Health Laboratory Services
NCHS	National Center for Health Statistics
NCI	National Cancer Institute
NCLEX-RN	National Council Licensure Examination for Registered Nurses
NCME	Network for Continuing Medical Education
NCMHD	National Center on Minority Health and Health Disparities (NIH)
NCMHI	National Clearinghouse for Mental Health Information
NCOA	National Council on Aging, Inc.
NCPIE	National Council on Patient Information and Education
NCRA	National Cancer Registrars Association
NCRP	National Council on Radiation Protection and Measurements

Abbreviation	Organization
NCRR	National Center for Research Resources (NIH)
NCTC	National Collection of Type Cultures
NCYC	National Collection of Yeast Cultures
NDA	National Dental Association
NDDG	National Diabetes Data Group
NDDIC	National Digestive Diseases Information Clearinghouse
NDIC	National Diabetes Information Clearinghouse
NDTI	National Disease and Therapeutic Index
NEHEP	National Eye Health Education Program
NEI	National Eye Institute
NEOPO	Northeast Organ Procurement Organization
NFB	National Foundation for the Blind
NFCA	National Family Caregivers Association
NGNA	National Gerontological Nursing Association
NHGRI	National Human Genome Research Institute (NIH)
NHIC	National Health Information Center
NHLBI	National Heart, Lung, and Blood Institute
NHPCO	National Hospice and Palliative Care Organization
NIA	National Institute on Aging (NIH)
NIAAA	National Institute on Alcohol Abuse and Alcoholism (NIH)
NIAID	National Institute of Acquired Immune Deficiency; National Institute of Allergy and Infectious Diseases (NIH)
NIAMS	National Institute of Arthritis and Musculoskeletal and Skin Diseases (NIH)
NIBIB	National Institute of Biomedical Imaging and Bioengineering
NICHD	National Institute of Child Health and Human Development

Abbreviation	Organization
NIDA	National Institute on Drug Abuse (NIH)
NIDCD	National Institute on Deafness and Other Communication Disorders
NIDCR	National Institute of Dental and Craniofacial Research
NIDDK	National Institute of Diabetes and Digestive and Kidney Disease
NIGMS	National Institute of General Medical Sciences (NIH)
NIH	National Institutes of Health
NIH-ORBD -NRC	NIH Osteoporosis and Related Bone Diseases National Resource Center
NIHR	National Institute for Healthcare Research
NIMH	National Institute of Mental Health (NIH)
NINDS	National Institute of Neurological Disorders and Stroke (NIH)
NIST	National Institute of Standards and Technology
NKF	National Kidney Foundation
NKUDIC	National Kidney and Urological Diseases Information Clearinghouse
NLHEP	National Lung Health Education Program
NLSBPH	National Library Service for the Blind and Physically Handicapped
NMA	National Medical Association
NMAC	National Medical Audiovisual Center
NMDP	National Marrow Donor Program
NMHA	National Mental Health Association
NMNRU	National Medical Neuropsychiatric Research Unit
NMSS	National Multiple Sclerosis Society
NNIS	National Nosocomial Infections Surveillance
NOF	National Osteoporosis Foundation
NORD	National Organization for Rare Disorders

Abbreviation	Organization
NOVS	National Office of Vital Statistics
NPCTG	National Prostatic Cancer Treatment Group
NPF	National Psoriasis Foundation
NPIN	National Prevention Information Network
NPTR	National Pediatric Trauma Registry
NRSCC	National Reference System in Clinical Chemistry
NSA	National Stroke Association
NSCIDRC	National Spinal Cord Injury Data Research Center
NSF	National Sleep Foundation
NTP	National Toxicology Program
NVAC	National Vaccine Advisory Committee
NWHIC	National Women's Health Information Center
NWHN	National Women's Health Network
OAA	Opticians Association of America
OAM	Office of Alternative Medicine
OCCAM	Office of Cancer Complementary and Alternative Medicine
OCD	Office of Child Development; Office of Civil Defense
OCHS	Office of Cooperative Health Statistics
OCIS	Oncology Center Information System
ODAC	Oncologic Drugs Advisory Committee (of the U.S. Food and Drug Administration)
ODSS	Office of Disability Support Services
OGD	Office of Generic Drugs (of the Food and Drug Administration)
OHTA	Office of Health Technology Assessment
OIF	Osteogenesis Imperfecta Foundation
OIG	Office of the Inspector General
OME	Office of the Medical Examiner
ONS	Oncology Nursing Society

Abbreviation	Organization
OPO	Organ Procurement Organization
OPTN	Organ Procurement and Transplantation Network
ORLAU	Orthotic Research and Locomotor Assessment Unit
OSH	Office on Smoking and Health
OSHA	Occupational Safety and Health Administration
OTIS	Organization of Teratology Information Services
OTOD	Organization of Teachers of Oral Diagnosis
OTSG	Office of the Surgeon General
OVR	Office of Vocational Rehabilitation
PAR	Program for Alcohol Recovery
PBA	Prevent Blindness America
PCC	Poison Control Center
PCPFS	President's Council on Physical Fitness and Sports
PDF	Parkinson's Disease Foundation
PFF	Pulmonary Fibrosis Foundation
PHTS	Pediatric Home Treatment Service
PLSG	Pigmented Lesion Study Group
PPFA	Planned Parenthood Federation of America
PRO	Peer Review Organization; Professional Review Organization
ProPAC	Prospective Payment Assessment Commission
PRSIS	Prospective Rate Setting Information System
PSEF	Plastic Surgery Educational Foundation
PSRC	Plastic Surgery Research Council
PSRO	Professional Standards Review Organization
RABBI	Rapid Access Blood Bank Information
RC	Red Cross
ROPA	Regional Organ Procurement Agency
RTECS	Registry of Toxic Effects of Chemical Substances

Abbreviation	Organization
SAGES	Society of American Gastrointestinal Endoscopic Surgeons
SAMHSA	Substance Abuse and Mental Health Services Administration
SART	Society for Assisted Reproductive Technology
SBH, SBOH	State Board of Health
SCHIP	State Children's Health Insurance Program
SHEA	Society for Healthcare Epidemiology of America
SIECUS	Sex Information and Educational Council of the United States
SIOP	International Society of Pediatric Oncology
SLICC	Systemic Lupus International Collaborating Clinics
SLT	Surgical Laser Technologies
SPP	Society for Pediatric Pathology
SSA	Social Security Administration
SSO	Society of Surgical Oncology
SSOP	Second Surgical Opinion Program
TCDB	Traumatic Coma Data Bank
TDB	Toxicology Data Bank
TERIS	Teratogen Information System
TIRR	The Institute for Rehabilitation Research
TMIC	Toxic Materials Information Center
UICC	International Union Against Cancer
UNOS	United Network for Organ Sharing
UOA	United Ostomy Association
USFDA	United States Food and Drug Administration
USH	United Services for Handicapped
USPHS	United States Public Health Service
USRDS	United States Renal Data System
VA	Department of Veterans Affairs
VEDA	Vestibular Disorders Association
VHA	Veterans Health Administration

Abbreviation	Organization
VIBS	Victims Information Bureau Service
VNA	Visiting Nurse Association
VNAA	Visiting Nurse Associations of America
VRS	Vocational Rehabilitation Services
WFC	World Federation of Chiropractic
WHO	World Health Organization
WHO/ILAR	World Health Organization/International League of Associations for Rheumatology

Healthcare Professional Designations

Abbreviation	Designation
AARCF	American Association for Respiratory Care Fellow
AAS	Associate in Applied Science
ACP	Advanced Clinical Practitioner
ADN	Associate Degree in Nursing
AHI	Allied Health Instructor (American Medical Technologists)
ANP	Adult Nurse Practitioner
APRN	Advance Practice Registered Nurse
APRN-BC	Advance Practice Registered Nurse-Board Certified
ARNP	Advanced Registered Nurse Practitioner
ART	Accredited Records Technologist
AT(ASCP)	Apheresis Technician (American Society for Clinical Pathology)
ATC	Athletic Trainer, Certified
AuD	Doctor of Audiology
BA	Bachelor of Arts
BB(ASCP)	Technologist in Blood Banking (American Society for Clinical Pathology)
BCCS	Board Certified in Clinical Social Work
BCNP	Board Certified Nuclear Pharmacist
BCNSP	Board Certified Nutrition Support Pharmacist
BCPS	Board Certified Pharmacotherapy Specialist
BS	Bachelor of Science
BSN	Bachelor of Science in Nursing
CADC	Certified Alcohol and Drug Counselor
CALN	Clinical Administrative Liaison Nurse

Abbreviation	Designation
C(ASCP)	Technologist in Chemistry (American Society for Clinical Pathology)
CAT(C)	Certified Athletic Therapist (Canada)
CCC-A	Certificate of Clinical Competence in Audiology
CCCP	Board Certified in Child and Adolescent Psychology
CCC-SLP	Certificate of Clinical Competence in Speech-Language Pathology
CCM	Certified Case Manager
CCMHC	Certified Clinical Mental Health Counselor
CCP	Certified Clinical Perfusionist
CCRN	Critical Care Registered Nurse
CCS	Cardiopulmonary Certified Specialist, Certified Coding Specialist
CDA	Certified Dental Assistant
CDE	Certified Diabetes Educator
CDT	Certified Dental Laboratory Technician
CEN	Certified Emergency Nurse
CCEMT-P	Critical Care Emergency Medical Technician– Paramedic
CCM	Certified Case Manager
CFNP	Certified Family Nurse Practitioner
CGT	Certified Gastroenterology Technician
CIH	Certificate in Industrial Health
CISW	Certified Independent Social Worker
CLA	Certified Laboratory Assistant
CLDir(NCA)	Clinical Laboratory Director (National Certification Agency for Medical Laboratory Personnel)
CLPlb(NCA)	Clinical Laboratory Phlebotomist (National Certification Agency for Medical Laboratory Personnel)

Abbreviation	Designation
CLS	Clinical Laboratory Scientist
CLS(NCA)	Clinical Laboratory Scientist (National Certification Agency for Medical Laboratory Personnel)
CLSp(CG)(NCA)	Clinical Laboratory Specialist in Cytogenetics (National Certification Agency for Medical Laboratory Personnel)
CLSp(H)(NCA)	Clinical Laboratory Specialist in Hematology (National Certification Agency for Medical Laboratory Personnel)
CLSup(NCA)	Clinical Laboratory Supervisor (National Certification Agency for Medical Laboratory Personnel)
CLT	Certified Laboratory Technician, Clinical Laboratory Technician
CLT(NCA)	Certified Laboratory Technician (National Certification Agency for Medical Laboratory Personnel)
CMA	Certified Medical Assistant
CMA-A	Certified Medical Assistant, Administrative
CMA-C	Certified Medical Assistant, Clinical
CMAS	Certified Medical Administrative Specialist (American Medical Technologists)
CMFT	Certified Marriage and Family Therapist
CMT	Certified Medical Transcriptionist (American Association for Medical Transcription)
CNA	Certified Nursing Assistant
CNIM	Certification in Neurophysiologic Intraoperative Monitoring (American Board of Registration of Electroencephalographic and Evoked Potential Technologists)
CNM	Certified Nurse Midwife

Abbreviation	Designation
CNMT	Certified Nuclear Medicine Technologist
CNOR	Certified Nurse Operating Room
CNP	Community Nurse Practitioner
CNS	Clinical Nurse Specialist
CNSD	Certified Nutrition Support Dietitian
CNSN	Certified Nutrition Support Nurse
CNSP	Certified Nutrition Support Physician
COLT	Certified Office Laboratory Technician (American Medical Technologists)
COMA	Certified Ophthalmic Medical Assistant
COMT	Certified Ophthalmic Medical Technologist
COTA	Certified Occupational Therapy Assistant (National Board for Certification in Occupational Therapy)
CP	Certified Psychologist, Clinical Psychologist
CPAN	Certified Post Anesthesia Nurse
CPFT	Certified Pulmonary Function Technologist (National Board of Respiratory Care)
CPH	Certificate in Public Health
CPN	Certified Pediatric Nurse
CPNP	Certified Pediatric Nurse Practitioner
CRNA	Certified Registered Nurse Anesthetist
CRTT	Certified Respiratory Therapy Technician
CSCS	Certified Strength and Conditioning Specialist
CST	Certified Surgical Technologist
CSW	Certified Social Worker, Clinical Social Worker
CT(ASCP)	Cytotechnologist (American Society for Clinical Pathology)
CTR	Certified Tumor Registrar

Abbreviation	Designation
CVO	Chief Veterinary Officer
CVT	Certified Veterinary Technician
CWOCN	Certified Wound, Ostomy, and Continence Nurse
DC	Doctor of Chiropractic
DDS	Doctor of Dental Surgery
DLM(ASCP)	Diplomate in Laboratory Management (American Society for Clinical Pathology)
DMD	Doctor of Dental Medicine
DME	Doctor of Medical Education
DMSc	Doctor of Medical Science
DNP	Doctor of Nursing Practice
DNS	Doctor of Nursing Science
DO	Doctor of Optometry (seen also as OD), Doctor of Osteopathy
DP	Doctor of Podiatry, Doctor of Pharmacy
DPH	Doctor of Public Health, Doctor of Public Hygiene
DPM	Doctor of Physical Medicine, Doctor of Podiatric Medicine
DPT	Doctor of Physical Therapy
DS	Doctor of Science
DSc	Doctor of Science
DSW	Doctor of Social Work
ECS (Clinical)	Electrophysiologic Certified Specialist (American Physical Therapists Association)
EdD	Doctor of Education
EFDA	Expanded Function Dental Auxiliary
EMT-B	Emergency Medical Technician–Basic (DOT classification; locales may vary)
EMT-D	Emergency Medical Technician–Defibrillation
EMT-I	Emergency Medical Technician–Intermediate (DOT classification; locales may vary)

Abbreviation	Designation
EMT-P	Emergency Medical Technician–Paramedic (DOT classification; locales may vary)
ENP	Emergency Nurse Practitioner
FAAMT	Fellow, American Association for Medical Transcription
FAAN	Fellow, American Academy of Nursing
FAARC	Fellow, American Association for Respiratory Care
FACD	Fellow, American College of Dentists
FACP	Fellow, American College of Physicians
FACS	Fellow, American College of Surgeons
FACSM	Fellow, American College of Sports Medicine
FADA	Fellow, American Dietetic Association
FAMA	Fellow, American Medical Association
FAOTA	Fellow, American Occupational Therapy Association
FAPTA	Fellow, American Physical Therapy Association
FCS	Fellow, College of Physicians and Surgeons
FFA	Fellow, Faculty of Anaesthetists (UK)
FFARCS	Fellow of the Faculty of Anaesthetists of the Royal College of Surgeons (UK)
FIAC	Fellow, International Academy of Cytology
FICC	Fellow of the International College of Chiropractors
FNAAOM	Fellow of the National Academy of Acupuncture and Oriental Medicine
FNP	Family Nurse Practitioner
FRCD	Fellow, Royal College of Dentists (UK)
FRCD(C)	Fellow, Royal College of Dentists of Canada
FRCGP	Fellow of the Royal College of General Practitioners

Abbreviation	Designation
FRCOG	Fellow of the Royal College of Obstetricians and Gynaecologists (UK)
FRCP	Fellow, Royal College of Physicians (UK)
FRCPA	Fellow, Royal College of Physicians of Australia
FRCPC	Fellow of the Royal College of Physicians of Canada
FRCPSC	Fellow, Royal College of Physicians and Surgeons of Canada
FRCR	Fellow of the Royal College of Radiologists
FRCS	Fellow of the Royal College of Surgeons (UK)
FRCSC	Fellow of the Royal College of Surgeons of Canada
FRS	Fellow of the Royal Society (Australia, Canada, Scotland, Ireland, UK)
FRSM	Fellow, Royal Society of Medicine (UK)
GCS	Geriatric Certified Specialist (American Physical Therapists Association)
GNP	Gerontological Nurse Practitioner
H(ASCP)	Technologist in Hematology (American Society for Clinical Pathology)
HP(ASCP)	Hemapheresis Practitioner (American Society for Clinical Pathology)
HT	Histotechnician (American Society for Clinical Pathology)
HTL(ASCP)	Histotechnologist (American Society for Clinical Pathology)
I(ASCP)	Technologist in Immunology (American Society for Clinical Pathology)
LAT	Licensed Athletic Trainer
LATC	Licensed Athletic Trainer, Certified

Abbreviation	Designation
LCSW	Licensed Clinical Social Worker
LD	Licensed Dietitian
LMCC	Licentiate of the Medical Council of Canada
LMFCC	Licensed Marriage, Family, and Child Counselor
LMP	Licensed Massage Practitioner
LMT	Licensed Massage Technician, Licensed Massage Therapist
LPN	Licensed Practical Nurse
LVN	Licensed Vocational Nurse
LVT	Licensed Veterinary Technician
MA	Master of Arts
M(ASCP)	Technologist in Microbiology (American Society for Clinical Pathology)
MB	Bachelor of Medicine
MBBS	Bachelor of Medicine (and) Bachelor of Surgery
MC	Master of Counseling
MCh	Master of Surgery
MD	Doctor of Medicine
ME	Medical Examiner
Med	Master of Education
MFC	Marriage and Family Counselor
MFCC	Marriage, Family, and Child Counselor
MFCT	Marriage, Family, and Child Therapist
MLT	Medical Laboratory Technician
MLT(ASCP)	Medical Laboratory Technician (American Society for Clinical Pathology)
MP(ASCP)	International Technologist in Molecular Pathology (American Society for Clinical Pathology)
MPH	Master of Public Health

Abbreviation	Designation
MPharm	Master in Pharmacy (Australia, New Zealand, UK, Ireland)
MPT	Master of Physical Therapy
MRCP	Member, Royal College of Physicians
MRCS	Member Royal College of Surgeons (UK)
MRL	Medical Records Librarian
MS	Master of Science, Master of Surgery
MSc	Master of Science
MSurg	Master of Surgery
MSN	Master of Science in Nursing
MSS	Master of Social Science
MSW	Medical Social Worker, Master of Social Work
MSSW	Master of Science in Social Work
MT	Medical Technologist (American Medical Technologists)
MT(ASCP)	Medical Technologist (American Society for Clinical Pathology)
MTA	Medical Technologist Assistant
NCC	National Certified Counselor
NCS	Neurologic Certified Specialist (American Physical Therapists Association)
NCTM	Nationally Certified in Therapeutic Massage (National Certification Board for Therapeutic Massage and Bodywork)
NCTMB	Nationally Certified in Therapeutic Massage and Bodywork (National Certification Board for Therapeutic Massage and Bodywork)
NM(ASCP)	Technologist in Nuclear Medicine (American Society for Clinical Pathology)
NMT	Nurse Massage Therapist, Nursing Massage Therapist
NP	Nurse Practitioner

Abbreviation	Designation
NREMT	National Registry Emergency Medical Technician–Basic or Candidate
NREMT-I	National Registry Emergency Medical Technician–Intermediate
NREMT-P	National Registry Emergency Medical Technician–Paramedic
OCS	Orthopedic Certified Specialist (American Physical Therapists Association)
OD	Doctor of Optometry (also seen as DO)
OT	Occupational Therapist
OT-C	Occupational Therapist (Canada)
OTD	Doctor of Occupational Therapy
OT/L	Occupational Therapist, Licensed
OTR	Occupational Therapist, Registered (National Board for Certification in Occupational Therapy)
PA	Physician's Assistant; Psychological Associate
PA-C	Physician Assistant–Certified
PA(ASCP)	Pathologists Assistant (American Society for Clinical Pathology)
PBT(ASCP)	Phlebotomy Technician (American Society for Clinical Pathology)
PCS	Pediatric Certified Specialist (American Physical Therapists Association)
PD	Doctor of Pharmacy
PharmD	Doctor of Pharmacy
PhD	Doctor of Philosophy
PhG	Graduate in Pharmacy (historic)
PNP	Pediatric Nurse Practitioner
PsyD	Doctor of Psychology
PT	Physical Therapist
PTA	Physical Therapy Assistant

Abbreviation	Designation
RD	Registered Dietitian
RDA	Registered Dental Assistant (American Medical Technologists)
RDCS	Registered Diagnostic Cardiac Sonographer (American Registry for Diagnostic Medical Sonography)
RDH	Registered Dental Hygienist
RDMS	Registered Diagnostic Medical Sonographer (American Registry for Diagnostic Medical Sonography)
RDN	Registered Dietitian/Nutritionist
R.EEGT	Registered Electroencephalographic Technologist (American Board of Registration of Electroencephalographic and Evoked Potential Technologists)
R.EPT.	Registered Evoked Potential Technologist (American Board of Registration of Electroencephalographic and Evoked Potential Technologists)
RHCP	Registered Health Care Provider
RHIA	Registered Health Information Administrator (American Health Information Management Association)
RHIT	Registered Health Information Technician (American Health Information Management Association)
RISW	Registered Independent Social Worker
RMA	Registered Medical Assistant (American Medical Technologists)
RMT	Registered Massage Therapist (Canada)
RN	Registered Nurse
RNCS	Registered Nurse Clinical Specialist

Abbreviation	Designation
RPFT	Registered Pulmonary Function Technologist (National Board of Respiratory Care)
RPh	Registered Pharmacist
RPSGT	Registered Polysomnographic Technologist (American Association of Sleep Technologists)
RPT	Registered Phlebotomy Technician (American Medical Technologists)
RPVT	Registered Physician in Vascular Interpretation (American Registry for Diagnostic Medical Sonography)
RRA	Registered Records Administrator
RRT	Registered Respiratory Therapist
RT	Radiologic Technologist; Respiratory Therapist
RT(ARRT)	Registered Technologist (American Registry of Radiologic Technologists)
RT(M)(AART)	Registered Technologist–Mammography (American Registry of Radiologic Technologists)
RT(N)(AART)	Registered Technologist–Nuclear Medicine (American Registry of Radiologic Technologists)
RT(R)	Technologist in Diagnostic Radiology
RTR	Registered Recreational Therapist
RT(T)(AART)	Registered Technologist–Radiation Therapy (American Registry of Radiologic Technologists)
RTT	Respiratory Therapy Technician
RVS	Registered Vascular Specialist
RVT	Registered Vascular Technologist (American Registry for Diagnostic Medical Sonography); Registered Veterinary Technician

Abbreviation	Designation
SAT	Supervisory Athletic Therapist (Canada)
SBB(ASCP)	Specialist in Blood Banking Technology (American Society for Clinical Pathology)
SC(ASCP)	Specialist in Chemistry (American Society for Clinical Pathology)
ScD	Doctor of Science
SCS	Sports Certified Specialist
SCT(ASCP)	Specialist in Cytotechnology (American Society for Clinical Pathology)
SH(ASCP)	Specialist in Hematology (American Society for Clinical Pathology)
SI(ASCP)	Specialist in Immunology (American Society for Clinical Pathology)
SL (ASCP)	Laboratory Safety Specialist (American Society for Clinical Pathology)
SLP	Speech-Language Pathologist
SM	Master of Surgery
SM(ASCP)	Specialist in Microbiology (American Society for Clinical Pathology)
SW	Social Worker
SV(ASCP)	Specialist in Virology (American Society for Clinical Pathology)
VTS	Veterinary Technician Specialist

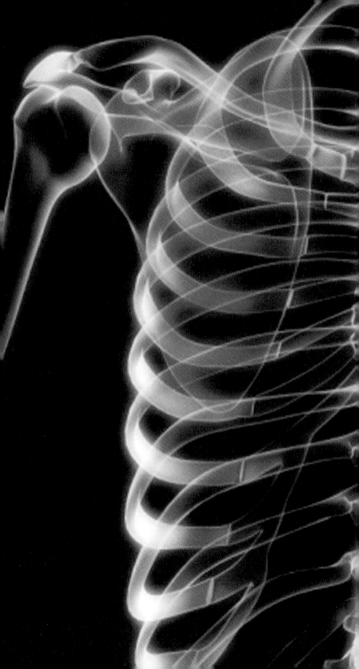

Body Planes

Figure 1.
Anatomical position with body planes.

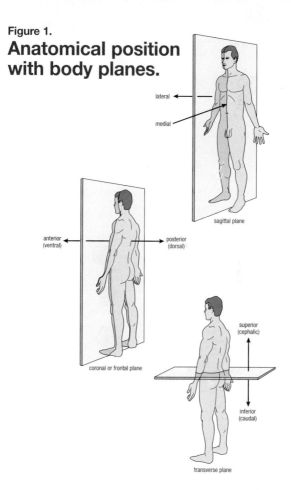

lateral

medial

sagittal plane

anterior
(ventral)

posterior
(dorsal)

coronal or frontal plane

superior
(cephalic)

inferior
(caudal)

transverse plane

Figure 2.
Anatomical position and directional references.

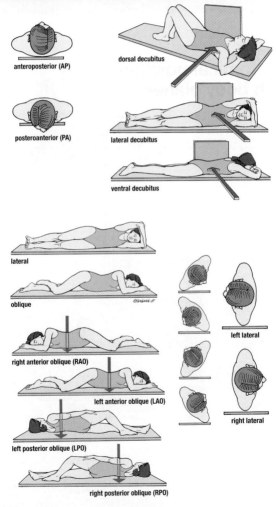

anteroposterior (AP)

posteroanterior (PA)

dorsal decubitus

lateral decubitus

ventral decubitus

lateral

oblique

right anterior oblique (RAO)

left anterior oblique (LAO)

left posterior oblique (LPO)

right posterior oblique (RPO)

left lateral

right lateral

Figure 3.
Positions on the operating table.

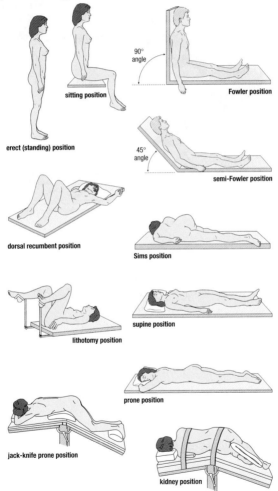

sitting position

Fowler position
90° angle

erect (standing) position

semi-Fowler position
45° angle

dorsal recumbent position

Sims position

lithotomy position

supine position

prone position

jack-knife prone position

kidney position

Figure 4.
Radiographic projections.

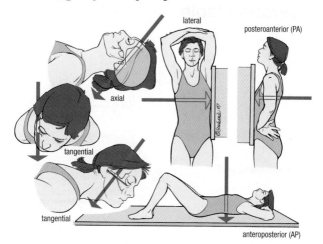

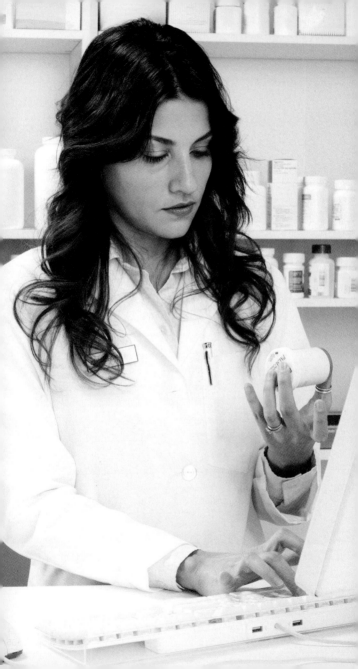

Pharmacology

Top 200 Commonly Prescribed Drugs

Drug	Manufacturer	Rank
Abilify (aripiprazole)	Otsuka	164
acetaminophen/codeine	Teva	68
AcipHex (rabeprazole)	Eisai	108
Actonel (risedronate)	Proctor & Gamble	61
Actos (pioglitazone)	Takeda	42
Adderall XR (dextroamphetamine/ amphetamine)	Shire	81
Advair Diskus (fluticasone/ salmeterol)	Glaxo SmithKline	20
albuterol	Armstrong	90
albuterol	Warrick	69
albuterol	Dey	157
allopurinol	Mylan	137
alprazolam	Sandoz	71
alprazolam	Greenstone	66
alprazolam	Mylan	128
alprazolam	Actavis	51
Altace (ramipril)	Monarch	54
Ambien (zolpidem)	Sanofi Aventis	91
Ambien CR (zolpidem)	Sanofi Aventis	79
amitriptyline hydrochloride	Mylan	138

Drug	Manufacturer	Rank
amlodipine besylate	Mylan	29
amlodipine besylate	Greenstone	93
amlodipine besylate/ benazepril	Teva	155
amoxicillin	Ranbaxy	64
amoxicillin	Teva	4
amoxicillin	Sandoz	151
amoxicillin trihydrate/ potassium clavulanate	Sandoz	80
amoxicillin trihydrate/ potassium clavulanate	Teva	139
Aricept (donepezil)	Eisai	73
atenolol	Sandoz	49
atenolol	Teva	144
atenolol	Mylan	40
Avandia (rosiglitazone)	Glaxo SmithKline	95
Avapro (irbesartan)	Bristol Myers	134
Avelox (moxifloxacin)	Schering Plough	190
azithromycin	Greenstone	13
azithromycin	Teva	41
azithromycin	Barr	172
Benicar (olmesartan)	Daiichi Sankyo	120
Benicar HCT (olmesartan/ hydrochlorothiazide)	Daiichi Sankyo	131
Boniva (ibandronate)	Roche	171
Budeprion XL (bupropion)	Teva	165
Cartia XT (diltiazem)	Watson	154
Celebrex (celecoxib)	Pfizer	47
cephalexin	Teva	28
Chantix (varenicline)	Pfizer	109
Cialis (tadalafil)	Lilly	162
ciprofloxacin hydrochloride	Rugby	163

Drug	Manufacturer	Rank
ciprofloxacin hydrochloride	Dr. Reddy	173
ciprofloxacin hydrochloride	Teva	177
citalopram hydrobromide	Aurobindo	186
clonazepam	Caraco	149
clonazepam	Teva	75
clonidine hydrochloride	Mylan	110
Combivent (ipratropium/ albuterol)	Boehringer Ingelheim	159
Concerta (methylphenidate)	McNeil	99
Coreg (carvedilol)	Glaxo SmithKline	77
Cozaar (losartan)	Merck	72
Crestor (rosuvastatin)	AstraZeneca	34
cyclobenzaprine hydrochloride	Barr	119
cyclobenzaprine hydrochloride	Mylan	129
Cymbalta (duloxetine)	Lilly	43
Depakote (valproic acid/ derivatives)	Abbott	188
Depakote ER (valproic acid/ derivatives)	Abbott	180
Detrol LA (tolterodine)	Pfizer	125
diazepam	Mylan	111
Digitek (digoxin)	Mylan	83
Diovan (valsartan)	Novartis	25
Diovan HCT (valsartan/ hydrochlorothiazide)	Novartis	39
doxycycline hyclate	Watson	142
Effexor XR (venlafaxine)	Wyeth	23
enalapril maleate	Mylan	178
Evista (raloxifene)	Lilly	156
fexofenadine hydrochloride	Teva	122

Drug	Manufacturer	Rank
fexofenadine hydrochloride	Prasco	136
fexofenadine hydrochloride	Dr. Reddy	148
Flomax (tamsulosin)	Boehringer Ingelheim	45
Flovent HFA (fluticasone (oral inhalation))	Glaxo SmithKline	176
fluconazole	Teva	127
fluoxetine hydrochloride	Barr	133
fluoxetine hydrochloride	Sandoz	189
fluoxetine hydrochloride	Teva	104
fluticasone propionate	Par	84
fluticasone propionate	Roxanne	118
Folic acid	Watson	183
Fosamax (alendronate)	Merck	26
furosemide	Mylan	19
furosemide	Teva	88
furosemide	Sandoz	117
gabapentin	Teva	85
glyburide	Teva	113
GlycoLax (polyethylene glycol 3350)	Kremers Urban	167
hydrochlorothiazide	Teva	18
hydrochlorothiazide	Qualitest	62
hydrochlorothiazide	Mylan	169
hydrocodone/acetaminophen	Mallinckrodt	2
hydrocodone/acetaminophen	Watson	3
hydrocodone/acetaminophen	Qualitest	78
Hyzaar (losartan/ hydrochlorothiazide)	Merck	114
ibuprofen (Rx)	Watson	94
ibuprofen (Rx)	Perrigo	184
ibuprofen (Rx)	Par	106
Imitrex (sumatriptan)	Glaxo SmithKline	146
isosorbide mononitrate	Ethex	140

Drug	Manufacturer	Rank
Klor-Con 10 (potassium chloride)	Upsher Smith	193
Klor-Con M20 (potassium chloride)	Upsher Smith	192
Lamictal (lamotrigine)	Glaxo SmithKline	98
Lantus (insulin glargine)	Sanofi Aventis	50
Levaquin (levofloxacin)	McNeil	37
Levothyroxine sodium	Mylan	5
Levothyroxine sodium	Lannett	30
Levothyroxine sodium	Sandoz	200
Levoxyl (levothyroxine)	King	70
Lexapro (escitalopram)	Forest	7
Lipitor (atorvastatin)	Pfizer	1
lisinopril	Sandoz	24
lisinopril	Mylan	160
lisinopril	Lupin	16
lisinopril	Teva	38
lisinopril/hydrochlorothiazide	Teva	197
lorazepam	Rugby	100
lorazepam	Watson	153
lorazepam	Sandoz	179
Lotrel (amlodipine/benazepril)	Novartis	82
lovastatin	Actavis	112
Lunesta (eszopiclone)	Sepacor	121
Lyrica (pregabalin)	Pfizer	92
meclizine hydrochloride	Par	199
metformin hydrochloride	Teva	35
metformin hydrochloride	Apotex	147
metformin hydrochloride	Zydus	166
methylprednisolone	Qualitest	191
metoprolol succinate	Par	74
metoprolol succinate	Sandoz	97

Drug	Manufacturer	Rank
metoprolol tartrate	Caraco	63
metoprolol tartrate	Mylan	31
Namenda (memantine)	Forest	135
Naproxen	Teva	130
Nasonex (mometasone)	Schering Plough	52
Nexium (esomeprazole)	AstraZeneca	9
Niaspan (niacin)	Abbott	170
Norvasc (amlodipine)	Pfizer	48
NuvaRing (ethinyl estradiol/etonogestrel)	Organon	187
omeprazole	Mylan	123
omeprazole	Sandoz	124
omeprazole	Apotex	132
omeprazole	Kremers Urban	198
Omnicef (cefdinir)	Abbott	181
Ortho Tri-Cy Lo 28 (ethinyl estradiol/norgestimate)	Ortho	103
oxycodone/acetaminophen	Watson	102
oxycodone/acetaminophen	Mallinckrodt	27
paroxetine hydrochloride	Apotex	76
penicillin V potassium	Teva	152
Plavix (clopidogrel)	Bristol Myers/Sanofi Aventis	11
potassium chloride	Ethex	107
potassium chloride	Teva	168
prednisone	Watson	44
prednisone	Roxane	182
Premarin (estrogens (conjugated/equine))	Wyeth	60
Prevacid (lansoprazole)	TAP	22
ProAir HFA (albuterol)	Teva	46
promethazine hydrochloride	Lilly	158

Drug	Manufacturer	Rank
propoxyphene-N/acetaminophen	Qualitest	55
propoxyphene-N/acetaminophen	Teva	143
Protonix (pantoprazole)	Wyeth	21
ranitidine hydrochloride	Teva	175
Requip (ropinirole)	Glaxo SmithKline	196
Risperdal (risperidone)	Jannsen	59
Seroquel (quetiapine)	AstraZeneca	36
sertraline hydrochloride	Greenstone	32
sertraline hydrochloride	Teva	56
simvastatin	Dr. Reddy	58
simvastatin	Teva	10
Singulair (montelukast)	Merck	8
Spiriva HandiHaler (tiotropium)	Boehringer Ingelheim	115
sulfamethoxazole/trimethoprim	Lannett	86
Synthroid (levothyroxine)	Abbott	6
Topamax (topiramate)	McNeil	96
Toprol-XL (metoprolol)	AstraZeneca	12
tramadol hydrochloride	Barr	185
tramadol hydrochloride	Teva	194
trazodone hydrochloride	Barr	57
triamterene/hydrochlorothiazide	Sandoz	89
triamterene/hydrochlorothiazide	Mylan	105
TriCor (fenofibrate)	Abbott	53
TriNessa-28 (ethinyl estradiol/norgestimate)	Watson	141

Drug	Manufacturer	Rank
Tri-Sprintec-28 (ethinyl estradiol/norgestimate)	Barr	195
Valtrex (valacyclovir)	Glaxo SmithKline	87
verapamil SR	Mylan	150
Viagra (sildenafil)	Pfizer	65
Vytorin (ezetimibe/ simvastatin)	Merck//Schering Plough	15
warfarin sodium	Barr	17
warfarin sodium	Taro	161
Wellbutrin XL (bupropion)	Glaxo SmithKline	116
Xalatan (latanoprost)	Pfizer	101
Yasmin 28 (ethinyl estradiol/ drospirenone)	Bayer	67
Yaz-28 (ethinyl estradiol/ drospirenone)	Bayer	174
Zetia (ezetimibe)	Merck//Schering Plough	33
zolpidem tartrate	Teva	126
Zyprexa (olanzapine)	Lilly	145
Zyrtec (cetirizine)	Pfizer	14

Source: Top 200 Prescription Drugs of 2007. *Pharmacy Times.* May 2008

Look-Alike and Sound-Alike Drug Names

Watch out for the following drug names that resemble other drug names, either in the way they are spelled or the way they sound.

Drug Name	Commonly Confused With
abciximab	infliximab
Accupril	Accutane
Acetazolamide	acetohexamide
Acetylcholine	acetylcysteine
Aciphex	Aricept
albuterol	atenolol or Albutein
Aldactone	Aldactazide
Aldomet	Aldoril or Anzemet
alitretinoin	tretinoin
amantadine	rimantadine
Ambien	Amen
Amicar	Amikin
amiloride	amiodarone
aminophylline	amitriptyline or ampicillin
Aminosyn	Amikacin
amiodarone	amiloride
amitriptyline	nortriptyline or aminophylline
amlodipine	amiloride
Anafranil	enalapril, nafarelin, or alfentanil
anakinra	amikacin
Anturane	Accutane or Artane
Anzemet	Aldomet
Apresoline	Apresazide
Aquasol A	AquaMEPHYTON

Drug Name	Commonly Confused With
Asacol	Os-Cal
Atarax	Ativan
atenolol	timolol or albuterol
Atrovent	Alupent
Avinza	Invanz
baclofen	Bactroban
Benadryl	Bentyl or Benylin
Bentyl	Aventyl or Benadryl and Proventil
benztropine	bromocriptine or brimonidine
Betagan	Betagen or Betapen-VK
Bumex	Buprenex
bupropion	buspirone
calcifediol	calcitriol
Carbatrol	carvedilol
carboplatin	cisplatin
Cardene	Cardura or codeine
Cardizem SR	Cardene SR
Cardura	Coumadin, K-Dur, Cardene, or Cordarone
Catapres	Cetapred or Combipres
Celebrex	Cerebyx or Celexa
Chloromycetin	chlorambucil
chlorpromazine	chlorpropamide
cimetidine	simethicone
clomiphene	clomipramine or clonidine
clonazepam	lorazepam
clonidine	quinidine or clomiphene
clorazepate	clofibrate
clotrimazole	co-trimoxazole
clozapine	Cloxapen, clofazimine, or Klonopin
codeine	Cardene, Lodine, or Cordran
Combivir	Epivir
corticotropin	cosyntropin

Drug Name	Commonly Confused With
Cozaar	Zocor and Hyzaar
cyclosporine	cycloserine
dacarbazine	Dicarbosil or procarbazine
Demerol	Demulen, Dymelor, or Temaril
desipramine	disopyramide or imipramine
desmopressin	vasopressin
desonide	Desogen or Desoxyn
dexamethasone	desoximetasone
Dexedrine	dextran or Excedrin
diazepam	diazoxide
diazoxide	Dyazide
diclofenac	Diflucan or Duphalac
dicyclomine	dyclonine or doxycycline
Dilantin	Dilaudid
dimenhydrinate	diphenhydramine
Diprivan	Ditropan
dipyridamole	disopyramide
dobutamine	dopamine
doxapram	doxorubicin, doxepin, or doxazosin
doxycycline	doxylamine or dicyclomine
dronabinol	droperidol
DynaCirc	Dynacin and Dynabac
Eldepryl	enalapril
enalapril	Anafranil or Eldepryl
epinephrine	ephedrine or norepinephrine
Epogen	Neupogen
Estratab	Estratest
ethosuximide	methsuximide
etidronate	etretinate, etidocaine, or etomidate
Eurax	Serax or Urex
fentanyl	alfentanil
Flexeril	Floxin or Flaxedil

Drug Name	Commonly Confused With
Flomax	Fosamax or Volmax
floxuridine	fludarabine or flucytosine
flunisolide	fluocinonide
fluorouracil	fludarabine, flucytosine, or floxuridine
fluoxetine	fluvoxamine or fluvastatin
fluticasone	fluconazole
folic acid	folinic acid
fosinopril	lisinopril
furosemide	torsemide
glimepiride	glyburide or glipizide
glucagon	Glaucon
guaifenesin	guanfacine
Haldol	Halcion or Halog
hydralazine	hydroxyzine
hydrocodone	hydrocortisone
hydromorphone	morphine
hydroxyzine	hydroxyurea or hydralazine
HyperHep	Hyperstat or Hyper-Tet
Hyperstat	Nitrostat
idarubicin	daunorubicin or doxorubicin
ifosfamide	cyclophosphamide
imipramine	desipramine
Imodium	Ionamin
Inderal	Inderide, Isordil, Adderall, or Imuran
Isoptin	Intropin
K-Phos-Neutral	Neutra-Phos-K
Lamictal	Lamisil
lamotrigine	lamivudine
Lanoxin	Levoxyl or levothyroxine
Lantus	Lente
Leukeran	leucovorin
Levatol	Lipitor

Drug Name	Commonly Confused With
levothyroxine	liothyronine or liotrix
Lithonate	Lithostat
Lithotabs	Lithobid or Lithostat
Lodine	codeine, iodine, or Iopidine
Lorabid	Lortab
lorazepam	alprazolam
Lotensin	Loniten or lovastatin
Luvox	Lasix
magnesium sulfate	manganese sulfate
Maxidex	Maxzide
Mestinon	Mesantoin or Metatensin
metaproterenol	metoprolol or metipranolol
methimazole	mebendazole or methazolamide
methocarbamol	mephobarbital
methylprednisolone	medroxyprogesterone
methyltestosterone	medroxyprogesterone
metoprolol	metaproterenol or metolazone
Mevacor	Mivacron
Micronor	Micro-K or Micronase
Minocin	niacin or Mithracin
mitomycin	mithramycin
Monopril	Monurol
naloxone	naltrexone
Navane	Nubain or Norvasc
Nicorette	Nordette
nifedipine	nimodipine or nicardipine
Nitro-Bid	Nicobid
nitroglycerine	nitroprusside
norepinephrine	epinephrine
Noroxin	Neurontin
nortriptyline	amitriptyline
Nubain	Navane
nystatin	Nitrostat

Drug Name	Commonly Confused With
Ocuflox	Ocufen
olsalazine	olanzapine
opium tincture	camphorated opium tincture
oxaprozin	oxazepam
oxymorphone	oxymetholone
pancuronium	pipecuronium
paroxetine	paclitaxel or pyridoxine
Paxil	Doxil, paclitaxel, or Taxol
pemoline	Pelamine
penicillamine	penicillin
penicillin G	Polycillin, penicillamine,
potassium	or other types of penicillin
pentobarbital	phenobarbital
pentostatin	pentosan
phentermine	phentolamine
phenytoin	mephenytoin
pindolol	Parlodel, Panadol, or Plendil
pioglitazone	rosiglitazone
Pitocin	Pitressin
pralidoxime	pramoxine or pyridoxine
Pravachol	Prevacid or propranolol
prednisolone	prednisone
Prilosec	Prozac, Prinivil, or Plendil
primidone	prednisone
Prinivil	Proventil or Prilosec
ProAmatine	protamine
probenecid	Procanbid
promethazine	promazine
ProSom	Proscar, Prozac, or Psorcon
protamine	Protopam or Protropin
pyridoxine	pralidoxime or Pyridium
Questran	Quarzan
quinidine	quinine or clonidine

Drug Name	Commonly Confused With
ranitidine	ritodrine or rimantadine
Reminyl	Robinul
Restoril	Vistaril
riboflavin	ribavirin
rifabutin	rifampin or rifapentine
Rifater	Rifadin or Rifamate
risperidone	reserpine
Ritalin	Rifadin
ritodrine	ranitidine
ritonavir	Retrovir
Sandimmune	Sandoglobulin or Sandostatin
saquinavir	saquinavir mesylate
Sarafem	Serophene
selegiline	Stelazine
Serentil	Serevent or Aventyl
Solu-Cortef	Solu-Medrol
somatropin	somatrem or sumatriptan
sotalol	Stadol
streptozocin	streptomycin
sufentanil	alfentanil or fentanyl
sulfadiazine	sulfasalazine
sulfamethoxazole	sulfamethizole
sulfasalazine	sulfisoxazole, salsalate, or sulfadiazine
sumatriptan	somatropin
Survanta	Sufenta
Tegretol	Toradol
Tenex	Xanax, Entex, or Ten-K
terbutaline	tolbutamide or terbinafine
terconazole	tioconazole
Testoderm	Estraderm
testosterone	testolactone
thiamine	Thorazine

Drug Name	Commonly Confused With
thioridazine	Thorazine
Tigan	Ticar
timolol	atenolol
Timoptic	Viroptic
tobramycin	Trobicin
Tobrex	Tobradex
tolnaftate	Tornalate
Toradol	Tegretol
Trental	Trendar or Trandate
triamcinolone	Triaminicin or Triaminicol
trifluoperazine	triflupromazine
trimipramine	triamterene or trimeprazine
Ultracet	Ultracef
Urispas	Urised
valacyclovir	valganciclovir
Vancenase	Vanceril
Vanceril	Vansil
Verelan	Vivarin, Ferralyn, or Virilon
Versed	VePesid
vidarabine	cytarabine
vinblastine	vincristine, vindesine, or vinorelbine
Volmax	Flomax
Voltaren	Ventolin or Verelan
Wellbutrin	Wellcovorin or Wellferon
Xanax	Zantac or Tenex
Xenical	Xeloda
Zarontin	Zaroxolyn
Zestril	Zostrix
Zocor	Zoloft
Zofran	Zosyn, Zantac, or Zoloft
Zyprexa	Zyrtec

Classification and Therapeutic Uses of Drugs

Classification of drugs is inherently difficult because many drugs can be classified in more than one way and some drugs do not fit well into any specific classification. Common ways to classify dugs include chemical (i.e., penicillins, opiates, thiazides), pharmacological (i.e., β-blockers, anticholinergics, antihistamines), and therapeutic (i.e., antiarrhythmics, antihypertensives, antidiabetics), among others. This list presents alternate classifications that drugs may belong to in addition to the listed classification. Finally, typical therapeutic uses are listed for each classification of drug, although this is not exhaustive and may not be representative of any particular drug in that group.

Classification	Alternate Classification(s)	Therapeutic Uses
α Blocker	α1 Adrenergic antagonist, antihypertensive, vasodilator	Hypertension, benign prostatic hyperplasia (BPH)
β Blocker	β Adrenergic antagonist, antihypertensive, antiarrhythmic, antianginal	Hypertension, cardiac arrhythmias, angina pectoris, congestive heart failure (CHF), migraine headache
β2 Agonist	β2 Adrenergic agonist, bronchodilator	Asthma, premature labor

Classification	Alternate Classification(s)	Therapeutic Uses
β-Lactamase inhibitor		β-Lactamase producing infection in combination with a β-lactamase susceptible penicillin
5α-Reductase inhibitor		Benign prostatic hyperplasia (BPH), alopecia
5-HT$_{1B/1D}$ agonist	Serotonin (5-hydroxytryptamine, 5-HT) 1B, 1D (5-HT$_{1B/1D}$) agonist, triptan	Migraine headache
5-HT$_3$ antagonist	Serotonin (5-hydroxytryptamine, 5-HT) 3 (5-HT$_3$) antagonist, antiemetic	Nausea, vomiting
5-HT$_4$ agonist	Serotonin (5-hydroxytryptamine, 5-HT) 4 (5-HT$_4$) agonist	Irritable bowel syndrome (IBS)
Aminoglycoside	Antimicrobial, antibacterial, antibiotic	Bacterial infections
Androgen	Anabolic steroid	Replacement therapy, cachexia
Angiotensin converting enzyme (ACE) inhibitor	Antihypertensive	Hypertension, congestive heart failure, diabetic renal nephropathy

Classification	Alternate Classification(s)	Therapeutic Uses
Angiotensin receptor blocker (ARB)	Antihypertensive	Hypertension, congestive heart failure
Antiandrogen		Prostate cancer
Antiarrhythmic		Cardiac arrhythmias
Antibacterial	Antimicrobial, antibiotic	Bacterial infections
Anticholinergic	Muscarinic antagonist	Parkinsonism, motion sickness, vertigo
Anticoagulant		Thromboembolic disorders
Anticonvulsant	Antiepileptic, antiseizure	Epilepsy, seizures, convulsions
Antiemetic		Nausea, vomiting
Antiestrogen		Estrogen dependent neoplastic disorders, infertility
Antifungal		Fungal infections
Antihistamine		Allergy, insomnia
Antimalarial		Malaria, nocturnal leg cramps (quinine)
Antimanic		Mania, bipolar disorder
Antineoplastic		Neoplastic disorders, immunological disorders
Antiprotozoal		Protozoal infections
Antipsychotic	Neuroleptic	Psychoses
Antithyroid		Hyperthyroidism

Classification	Alternate Classification(s)	Therapeutic Uses
Antiviral		Viral infections
Anxiolytic		Anxiety
Atypical antidepressant		Major depressive disorder
Atypical antipsychotic	Neuroleptic	Psychoses
Barbiturate	Sedative, hypnotic, general anesthetic, central nervous system (CNS) depressant, anticonvulsant, anxiolytic	Insomnia, epilepsy, seizures, convulsions, anxiety, general anesthesia
Benzodiazepine	Sedative, hypnotic, central nervous system (CNS) depressant, anticonvulsant, anxiolytic	Insomnia, epilepsy, seizures, convulsions, anxiety
Benzodiazepine receptor agonist	Sedative, hypnotic	Insomnia
Bile acid sequestrant		Hyperlipidemia, hypercholesterolemia
Bisphosphonate	Bone resorption inhibitor	Paget disease, osteoporosis, hypercalcemia
Calcium channel blocker	Slow channel blocker, antihypertensive, antiarrhythmic, antianginal	Hypertension, cardiac arrhythmias, angina pectoris

Classification	Alternate Classification(s)	Therapeutic Uses
Carbonic anhydrase inhibitor	Diuretic	Edema, epilepsy, glaucoma
Cardiac glycoside	Inotropic	Congestive heart failure (CHF), supraventricular tachycardia
Cardioselective β blocker	β_1 Adrenergic antagonist, antihypertensive, antiarrhythmic, antianginal	Hypertension, cardiac arrhythmias, angina pectoris, congestive heart failure (CHF)
Central nervous system (CNS) stimulant		Attention deficit-hyperactivity disorder (ADHD), obesity
Central sympatholytic	α_2 Adrenergic agonist, antihypertensive	Hypertension, skeletal muscle spasms
Cephalosporin	Antimicrobial, antibacterial, antibiotic	Bacterial infections
Cholesterol absorption inhibitor		Hypercholesterolemia
Cholinesterase inhibitor	Acetylcholinesterase inhibitor, cholinergic, parasympathomimetic	Myasthenia gravis, Alzheimer disease
Combination product	See individual ingredients	See individual ingredients

Classification	Alternate Classification(s)	Therapeutic Uses
COX2 Inhibitor	Cyclooxygenase-2 (COX2) Inhibitor, nonsteroidal anti-inflammatory drug (NSAID), analgesic, antiinflammatory, antipyretic	Pain, inflammation, fever, arthritis
Cytoprotective		Peptic ulcer disease (PUD)
Disease-modifying antirheumatic drug (DMARD)	Immune response modifier, biologic response modifier, immunomodulator	Rheumatoid arthritis, immunological disorders
DOPA decarboxylase inhibitor	Dihydroxyphenyla-lanine (DOPA) decarboxylase inhibitor	Parkinsonism (only with levodopa)
Dopaminergic		Parkinsonism, galactorrhea (Commonly used in combination with a progestin)
Estrogen	Oral contraceptive, birth control pills	Contraception, menstrual irregularities, infertility, menopause, replacement therapy, vaginal atrophy, osteoporosis, ovarian failure

Classification	Alternate Classification(s)	Therapeutic Uses
Expectorant		Cough
Fibric acid derivative		Hyperlipidemia, hypertriglyceridemia, hypercholesterolemia
Fluoroquinolone	Quinolone	Bacterial infections
Gallstone solubilizing agent	Gallstone dissolution agent	Gallstones
Ganglionic stimulant		Smoking cessation
Glucocorticoid	Steroid, corticosteroid, adrenocortical steroid, immunosuppressant	Inflammation, immunological disorders, allergies
Granulocyte colony stimulating factor (G-CSF)		Decrease infections during myelosuppressive treatment
H_2 receptor antagonist (H_2RA)	Histamine H_2 receptor antagonist (H_2RA), H_2 blocker	Peptic ulcer disease (PUD), gastroesophageal reflux disease (GERD)
Histamine analog		Ménière disease
HMG-CoA reductase inhibitor	Statin	Hyperlipidemia, hypercholesterolemia
Hydantoin	Anticonvulsant, antiepileptic, antiseizure	Epilepsy, seizures, convulsions

Classification	Alternate Classification(s)	Therapeutic Uses
Immunomodulator	Immune response modifier, biologic response modifier	Immunological disorders, viral infections, neoplastic disorders
Immuno-suppressant		Immunological disorders, autoimmune disorders, organ and tissue transplants (allografts)
Indirect-acting sympathomimetic	Anorexiant, decongestant, central nervous system (CNS) stimulant	Nasal congestion, obesity, attention deficit–hyperactivity disorder (ADHD)
Insulin	Antidiabetic	Type I and Type II diabetes mellitus
Keratolytic		Acne vulgaris, UV damaged skin, wart removal
Laxative		Constipation, bowel evacuation
Lincosamide	Antimicrobial, antibacterial, antibiotic	Bacterial infections
Local anesthetic		Pain
Loop diuretic		Edema, congestive heart failure (CHF), renal failure, hypertension

Classification	Alternate Classification(s)	Therapeutic Uses
Low molecular weight heparin (LMWH)	Anticoagulant, antithrombic	Thromboembolic disorders
LTD_4 receptor antagonist	Leukotriene D_4 (LTD_4) receptor antagonist	Asthma
Macrolide	Antimicrobial, antibacterial, antibiotic	Bacterial infections
Methylxanthine	Bronchodilator, central nervous system (CNS) stimulant	Asthma, apnea of prematurity, drowsiness
Nitrate	Vasodilator, venodilator, antianginal	Angina pectoris, hypertension
Nonsteroidal antiinflammatory drug (NSAID)	Analgesic, anti-inflammatory, antipyretic	Pain, inflammation, fever
Opiate agonist	Analgesic, narcotic, opioid, antitussive, antidiarrheal	Pain, cough, diarrhea
Oral antidiabetic	Oral hypoglycemic	Type II diabetes mellitus
Penicillin	Antimicrobial, antibacterial, antibiotic	Bacterial infections
Phenothiazine	Antipsychotic, antiemetic, antihistamine	Psychoses, nausea, vomiting, allergies

Classification	Alternate Classification(s)	Therapeutic Uses
Phosphate binder		Reduce intestinal absorption of phosphate in renal failure
Phosphodiesterase type 5 (PDE5) inhibitor		Erectile dysfunction (ED)
Platelet aggregation inhibitor		Prevention of myocardial infarction
Potassium sparing diuretic		Hypertension, edema, offset potassium loss of potassium depleting diuretics (thiazide and loop diuretics)
Progestin	Oral contraceptive, birth control pills	(Commonly used in combination with an estrogen) Contraception, menstrual irregularities, infertility, menopause, replacement therapy, vaginal atrophy, osteoporosis, ovarian failure
Prokinetic		Gastroparesis, gastroesophageal reflux disease (GERD)

Classification	Alternate Classification(s)	Therapeutic Uses
Prostaglandin		Peptic ulcer disease (PUD), glaucoma, erectile dysfunction (ED), cervical dilatation
Protease inhibitor	Antiretroviral, antiviral	Human immunodeficiency virus (HIV) infection
Proton pump inhibitor (PPI)		Peptic ulcer disease (PUD), gastroesophageal reflux disease (GERD)
Recombinant human erythropoietin		Anemia
Retinoid		Acne
Reverse transcriptase inhibitor	Antiretroviral, antiviral	Human immunodeficiency virus (HIV) infection
Selective estrogen receptor modulator (SERM)	Estrogen agonist/antagonist	Osteoporosis, infertility
Selective norepinephrine reuptake inhibitor (SNRI)	Antidepressant	Major depressive disorder
Selective serotonin reuptake inhibitor (SSRI)	Antidepressant	Major depressive disorder

Classification	Alternate Classification(s)	Therapeutic Uses
Skeletal muscle relaxant		Skeletal muscle spasms and spasticity
Stool softener		Constipation
Sulfonamide	Antimicrobial, antibacterial, antibiotic	Bacterial infections
Tetracycline	Antimicrobial, antibacterial, antibiotic	Bacterial, rickettsial, chlamydial infections
Thiazide and related diuretics	Antihypertensive	Edema, hypertension
Thyroid hormone		Hypothyroidism
Tricyclic antidepressant (TCA)	Antidepressant	Major depressive disorder
Urinary analgesic		Urinary tract pain
Vasodilator	Antihypertensive	Hypertension, peripheral vascular diseases
Vasopressin analog		Replacement therapy, nocturnal enuresis
Xanthine oxidase inhibitor		Gout

Error-Prone Pharmaceutical Abbreviations, Symbols, and Dose Designations

Error-Prone Pharmaceutical Abbreviations

The abbreviations, symbols, and dose designations found in these tables have been reported to the Institute for Safe Medication Practices (ISMP; www.ismp.org) through the USP-ISMP Medication Error Reporting Program as being frequently misinterpreted and involved in harmful medication errors. They should never be used when communicating medical information. This includes internal communications, telephone/verbal prescriptions, computer-generated labels, labels for drug storage bins, medication administration records, as well as pharmacy and prescriber computer order entry screens.

The Joint Commission has established a National Patient Safety Goal that specifies that certain abbreviations must appear on an accredited organization's do-not-use list; we have highlighted these items with an asterisk (*). However, we hope that you will consider others beyond the minimum Joint Commission requirements. By using and promoting safe practices and by educating one another about hazards, we can better protect our patients.

ISMP's Error-Prone Pharmaceutical Abbreviations

Abbreviation	Intended Meaning	Misinterpretation	Correction
μg	Microgram	Mistaken as "mg"	Use "mcg"
AD, AS, AU	Right ear, left ear, each ear	Mistaken as OD, OS, OU (right eye, left eye, each eye)	Use "right ear," "left ear," or "each ear"
OD, OS, OU	Right eye, left eye, each eye	Mistaken as AD, AS, AU (right ear, left ear, each ear)	Use "right eye," "left eye," or "each eye"
BT	Bedtime	Mistaken as "BID" (twice daily)	Use "bedtime"
cc	Cubic centimeters	Mistaken as "u" (units)	Use "mL"
D/C	Discharge or discontinue	Premature discontinuation of medications if D/C (intended to mean "discharge") has been misinterpreted as "discontinued" when followed by a list of discharge medications	Use "discharge" and "discontinue"
IJ	Injection	Mistaken as "IV" or "intrajugular"	Use "injection"
IN	Intranasal	Mistaken as "IM" or "IV"	Use "intranasal" or "NAS"

Abbreviation	Intended Meaning	Misinterpretation	Correction
HS	Half-strength	Mistaken as bedtime	Use "half-strength" or "bedtime"
hs	At bedtime, hours of sleep	Mistaken as half-strength	Use "half-strength" or "bedtime"
IU*	International unit	Mistaken as IV (intravenous) or 10 (ten)	Use "units"
o.d. or OD	Once daily	Mistaken as "right eye" (OD-oculus dexter), leading to oral liquid medications administered in the eye	Use "daily"
OJ	Orange juice	Mistaken as OD or OS (right or left eye); drugs meant to be diluted in orange juice may be given in the eye	Use "orange juice"
Per os	By mouth, orally	The "os" can be mistaken as "left eye" (OS-oculus sinister)	Use "PO," "by mouth," or "orally"
q.d. or QD*	Every day	Mistaken as q.i.d., especially if the period after the "q" or the tail of the	Use "daily"

Abbreviation	Intended Meaning	Misinterpretation	Correction
		"q" is misunderstood as an "i"	
qhs	Nightly at bedtime	Mistaken as "qhr" or every hour	Use "nightly"
qn	Nightly or at bedtime	Mistaken as "qh" (every hour)	Use "nightly" or "at bedtime"
q.o.d. or QOD*	Every other day	Mistaken as "q.d. (daily) or "q.i.d. (four times daily) if the "o" is poorly written	Use "every other day"
qld	Daily	Mistaken as q.i.d. (four times daily)	Use "daily"
q6PM, etc.	Every evening at 6 PM	Mistaken as every 6 hours	Use "6 PM nightly" or "6 PM daily"
SC, SQ, sub q	Subcutaneous	SC mistaken as SL (sublingual); SQ mistaken as "5 every;" the "q" in "sub q" has been mistaken as "every" (e.g., a heparin dose ordered "sub q 2 hours before	Use "subcut" or "subcutaneously"

Abbreviation	Intended Meaning	Misinterpretation	Correction
		surgery" misunderstood as every 2 hours before surgery)	
ss	Sliding scale (insulin) or ½ (apothecary)	Mistaken as "55"	Spell out "sliding scale;" use "one-half" or "½"
SSRI	Sliding scale regular insulin	Mistaken as selective-serotonin reuptake inhibitor	Spell out "sliding scale (insulin)"
SSI	Sliding scale insulin	Mistaken as Strong Solution of Iodine (Lugol's)	
i/d	One daily	Mistaken as "tid"	Use "1 daily"
TIW or tiw	3 times a week	Mistaken as "3 times a day" or "twice in a week"	Use "3 times weekly"
U or u*	Unit	Mistaken as the number 0 or 4, causing a 10-fold overdose or greater (e.g., 4U seen as "40" or 4u seen as "44"); mistaken as "cc" so dose given in volume instead of units (e.g., 4u seen as 4cc)	Use "unit"

Error-Prone Dose Designations and Other Information

Dose Designation	Intended Meaning	Misinterpretation	Correction
Trailing zero after decimal point (eg, 1.0 mg)*	1 mg	Mistaken as 10 mg if the decimal point is not seen	Do not use trailing zeros for doses expressed in whole numbers
"Naked" decimal point (eg, .5 mg)*	0.5 mg	Mistaken as 5 mg if the decimal point is not seen	Use zero before a decimal point when the dose is less than a whole unit
Drug name and dose run together (especially problematic for drug names that end in "l" such as Inderal 40 mg; Tegretol 300 mg)	Inderal 40 mg Tegretol 300 mg	Mistaken as Inderal 140 mg Mistaken as Tegretol 1300 mg	Place adequate space between the drug name, dose, and unit of measure

Dose Designation	Intended Meaning	Misinterpretation	Correction
Numerical dose and unit of measure run together (eg, 10mg, 100mL)	10 mg 100 mL	The "m" is sometimes mistaken as a zero or two zeros, risking a 10- to 100-fold overdose	Place adequate space between the dose and unit of measure
Abbreviations such as mg. or mL. with a period following the abbreviation	mg mL	The period is unnecessary and could be mistaken as the number 1 if written poorly	Use mg, mL, etc. without a terminal period
Large doses without properly placed commas (e.g., 100000 units; 1000000 units)	100,000 units 1,000,000 units	100000 has been mistaken as 10,000 or 1,000,000; 1000000 has been mistaken as 100,000	Use commas for dosing units at or above 1,000, or use words such as 100 "thousand" or 1 "million" to improve readability

Error-Prone Drug Name Abbreviations

Abbreviation	Intended Meaning	Misinterpretation	Correction
ARA A	vidarabine	Mistaken as cytarabine (ARA C)	Use complete drug name
AZT	zidovudine (Retrovir)	Mistaken as azathioprine or aztreonam	Use complete drug name
CPZ	Compazine (prochlorperazine)	Mistaken as chlorpromazine	Use complete drug name
DPT	Demerol-Phenergan-Thorazine	Mistaken as diphtheria-pertussis-tetanus (vaccine)	Use complete drug name
DTO	Diluted tincture of opium, or deodorized tincture of opium (Paregoric)	Mistaken as tincture of opium	Use complete drug name
HCl	hydrochloric acid or hydrochloride	Mistaken as potassium chloride (The "H" is misinterpreted as "K")	Use complete drug name unless expressed as a salt of a drug
HCT	hydrocortisone	Mistaken as hydrochlorothiazide	Use complete drug name

Abbreviation	Intended Meaning	Misinterpretation	Correction
HCTZ	hydrochlorot-hiazide	Mistaken as hydro-cortisone (seen as HCT250 mg)	Use complete drug name
"IV Vanc"	intravenous vancomycin	Mistaken as Invanz	Use complete drug name
MgSO4*	magnesium sulfate	Mistaken as morphine sulfate	Use complete drug name
MS, MSO4*	morphine sulfate	Mistaken as magnesium sulfate	Use complete drug name
MTX	methotre-xate	Mistaken as mitoxantrone	Use complete drug name
"Nitro" drip	nitroglycerin infusion	Mistaken as sodium nitro-prusside infusion	Use complete drug name
"Norflox"	norfloxacin	Mistaken as Norflex	Use complete drug name
PCA	procaina-mide	Mistaken as patient controlled analgesia	Use complete drug name
PTU	propylthi-ouracil	Mistaken as mercaptopurine	Use complete drug name
T3	Tylenol with codeine No. 3	Mistaken as liothyronine	Use complete drug name

Abbreviation	Intended Meaning	Misinterpretation	Correction
TAC	triamcinol-one	Mistaken as tetracaine, Adrenalin, cocaine	Use complete drug name
TNK	TNKase	Mistaken as "TPA"	Use complete drug name
ZnSO4	zinc sulfate	Mistaken as morphine sulfate	Use complete drug name

Error-Prone Pharmaceutical Symbols

Symbol	Intended Meaning	Misinterpretation	Correction
℥	Dram	Symbol for dram mistaken as "3"	Use the metric system
	Minim	Symbol for minim mistaken as "mL"	
×3d	For three days	Mistaken as "3 doses"	Use "for three days"
> and <	Greater than and less than	Mistaken as opposite of intended; mistakenly use incorrect symbol; "< 10" mistaken as "40"	Use "greater than" or "less than"
/ (slash mark)	Separates two doses or indicates "per"	Mistaken as the number 1 (e.g., "25 units/10 units" misread as "25 units and 110" units)	Use "per" rather than a slash mark to separate doses
@	At	Mistaken as "2"	Use "at"
&	And	Mistaken as "2"	Use "and"
+	Plus or and	Mistaken as "4"	Use "and"
°	Hour	Mistaken as a zero (e.g., q2° seen as q 20)	Use "hr," "h," or "hour"

Source: Error-Prone Abbreviation List. Institute for Safe Medication Practices. Available at: http://www.ismp.org/Tools/errorproneabbreviations.pdf. Accessed June 10, 2008.

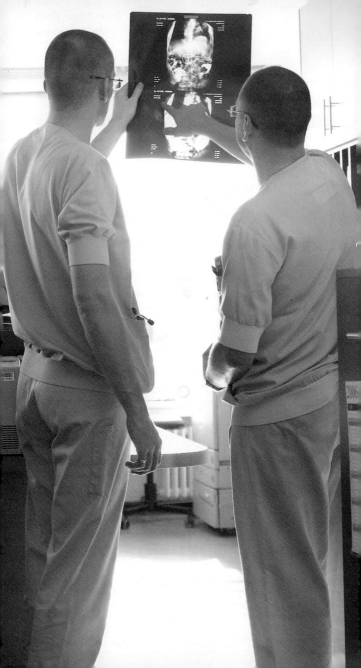

Laboratory and Diagnostic Information

Laboratory Values

Tests	Conventional Units	SI Units
Acetaminophen, serum or plasma (Hep or EDTA)		
Therapeutic	10–30 mcg/mL	66–199 mcmol/L
Toxic	>200 mcg/mL	>1324 mcmol/L
Acetone		
Serum		
Qualitative	Negative	Negative
Quantitative	0.3–2.0 mg/dL	0.05–0.34 mmol/L
Urine		
Qualitative	Negative	Negative
Acid hemolysis test (Ham)	<5% lysis	<0.05 lysed fraction
Adrenocorticotropin (ACTH), plasma		
8 AM	<120 pg/mL	<26 pmol/L
Midnight (supine)	<10 pg/mL	<2.2 pmol/L
Alanine aminotransferase (ALT, SGPT), serum*		
Male	13–40 U/L (37°C)	0.22–0.68 mckat/L (37°C)
Female	10–28 U/L (37°C)	0.17–0.48 mckat/L (37°C)

Tests	Conventional Units	SI Units
Albumin		
Serum		
Adult	3.5–5.2 g/dL	35–52 g/L
	3.2–4.6 g/dL	32–46 g/L
>60 years	Average of 0.3 g/dL higher in patients in upright position	Average of 3 g/L higher in patients in upright position
Urine		
Qualitative	Negative	Negative
Quantitative	50–80 mg/24 h	50–80 mg/24 h
CSF	10–30 mg/dL	100–300 mg/L
Aldolase, serum*	1.0–7.5 U/L (30° C)	0.02–0.13 mckat/L (30° C)
Aldosterone		
Serum		
Supine	3–16 ng/dL	0.08–0.44 nmol/L
Standing	7–30 ng/dL	0.19–0.83 nmol/L
Urine	3–19 mcg/24 h	8–51 nmol/24 h
Amikacin, serum or plasma (EDTA)		
Therapeutic		
Peak	25–35 mcg/mL	43–60 mcmol/L
Trough		
Less severe infection	1–4 mcg/mL	1.7–6.8 mcmol/L
Life-threatening infection	4–8 mcg/mL	6.8–13.7 mcmol/L
Toxic		
Peak	>35–40 mcg/mL	>60–68 mcmol/L
Trough	>10–15 mcg/mL	>17–26 mcmol/L

Tests	Conventional Units	SI Units
∂-Aminolevulinic acid, urine	1.3–7.0 mg/ 24 h	10–53 mcmol/ 24 h
Amitriptyline, serum or plasma (Hep or EDTA); trough (≥12 h after dose)		
Therapeutic	80–250 ng/mL	289–903 nmol/L
Toxic	>500 ng/mL	>1805 nmol/L
Ammonia		
Plasma (Hep)	9–33 mcmol/L	9–33 mcmol/L
Amylase*		
Serum	27–131 U/L	0.46–2.23 mckat/L
Urine	1–17 U/h	0.017–0.29 mckat/h
Amylase:creatinine clearance ratio	1–4%	0.01–0.04
Androstenedione, serum		
Male	75–205 ng/dL	2.6–7.2 nmol/L
Female	85–275 ng/dL	3.0–9.6 nmol/L
Anion gap		
(Na – [Cl + HCO_3])	7–16 mEq/L	7–16 mmol/L
([Na + K] – [Cl + HCO_3])	10–20 mEq/L	10–20 mmol/L
α1-Antitrypsin, serum	78–200 mg/dL	0.78–2.00 g/L
Apolipoprotein A-1		
Male	94–178 mg/dL	0.94–1.78 g/L
Female	101–199 mg/dL	1.01–1.99 g/L
Apolipoprotein B		
Male	63–133 mg/dL	0.63–1.33 g/L
Female	60–126 mg/dL	0.60–1.26 g/L

Tests	Conventional Units	SI Units
Arsenic		
Whole blood (Hep)	0.2–2.3 mcg/dL	0.03–0.31 mcmol/L
Chronic poisoning	10–50 mcg/dL	1.33–6.65 mcmol/L
Acute poisoning	60–930 mcg/dL	7.98–124 mcmol/L
Urine, 24 h	5–50 mcg/d	0.07–0.67 mcmol/d
Ascorbic acid, plasma (Ox, Hep, EDTA)	0.4–1.5 mg/dL	23–85 mcmol/L
Aspartate aminotransferase (AST, SGOT), serum*	10–59 U/L (37°C)	0.17–1.00 −2 to +3 kat/L (37°C)
Base excess, blood (Hep)	−2 to +3 mEq/L	22 to +3 mmol/L
Bicarbonate, serum (venous)	22–29 mEq/L	22–29 mmol/L
Bilirubin*†		
Bilirubin, direct		
Birth–death	0.0–0.4 mg/dL	
Bilirubin, total		
Birth–1 day	1.0–6.0 mg/dL	
1–2 days	6.0–7.5 mg/dL	
2–5 days	4.0–13.5 mg/dL	
5 days–death	0.2–1.2 mg/dL	
Total bilirubin, neonatal		
Birth–1 day	1.0–6.0 mg/dL	
1–2 days	6.0–7.5 mg/dL	
2–5 days	4.0–13.5 mg/dL	

Tests	Conventional Units	SI Units
5 days– 1 month	0.0–1.8 mg/dL	
1 month– death	0.0–1.8 mg/dL	
Bone marrow, differential cell count		
Adult		
Undifferentiated cells	0–1%	0–0.01
Myeloblast	0–2%	0–0.02
Promyelocyte	0–4%	0–0.04
Myelocytes		
Neutrophilic	5–20%	0.05–0.20
Eosinophilic	0–3%	0–0.03
Basophilic	0–1%	0–0.01
Metamyelocytes and bands		
Neutrophilic	5–35%	0.05–0.35
Eosinophilic	0–5%	0–0.05
Basophilic	0–1%	0–0.01
Segmented neutrophils	5–15%	0.05–0.15
Pronormoblast	0–1.5%	0–0.015
Basophilic normoblast	0–5%	0–0.05
Polychromato-philic normoblast	5–30%	0.05–0.30
Orthochromatic normoblast	5–10%	0.05–0.10
Lymphocytes	10–20%	0.10–0.20
Plasma cells	0–2%	0–0.02
Monocytes	0–5%	0–0.05

Tests	Conventional Units	SI Units
CA-125, serum	<35 U/mL	<35 kU/L
CA 15-3, serum	<30 U/mL	<30 kU/L
CA 19-9, serum	<37 U/mL	<37 kU/L
Cadmium, whole blood (Hep)	0.1–0.5 mcg/dL	8.9–44.5 nmol/L
Toxic	10–300 mcg/dL	0.89–26.70 mcmol/L
Cadmium, urine, 24 h	<15 mcg/d	<0.13 mcmol/d
Calcitonin, serum or plasma		
Male	≤100 pg/mL	≤100 ng/L
Female	≤30 pg/mL	≤30 ng/L
Calcium, serum	8.6–10.0 mg/dL (slightly higher in children)	2.15–2.50 mmol/L (slightly higher in children)
Calcium, ionized, serum	4.64–5.28 mg/dL	1.16–1.32 mmol/L
Calcium, urine		
Low calcium diet	50–150 mg/24 h	1.25–3.75 mmol/24 h
Usual diet; trough	100–300 mg/24 h	2.50–7.50 mmol/24 h
Carbamazepine, serum or plasma (Hep or EDTA), trough		
Therapeutic	4–12 mcg/mL	17–51 mcmol/L
Toxic	>15 mcg/mL	>63 mcmol/L

Tests	Conventional Units	SI Units
Carbon dioxide, total, serum/ plasma (Hep)	22–28 mmol/L	22–28 mmol/L
Carbon dioxide (PCO_2), blood, arterial	Male 35–48 mmHg Female 32–45 mmHg	4.66–6.38 kPa 4.26–5.99 kPa
Carbon monoxide as carboxyhemoglobin (HbCO), whole blood (EDTA)		
Nonsmokers	0.5–1.5% total Hb	0.005–0.015 HbCO fraction
Smokers		
1–2 packs/d	4–5% total Hb	0.04–0.05 HbCO fraction
> 2 packs/d	8–9% total Hb	0.08–0.09 HbCO fraction
Toxic	>20% total Hb	>0.20 HbCO fraction
Lethal	>50% total Hb	>0.5 HbCO fraction
Carotene, serum	10–85 mcg/dL	0.19–1.58 mcmol/L
Catecholamines, plasma (EDTA)		
Dopamine	<30 pg/mL	<196 pmol/L
Epinephrine	<140 pg/mL	<764 pmol/L
Norepinephrine	<1700 pg/mL	<10,047 pmol/L
Catecholamines, urine		
Dopamine	65–400 mcg/24 h	425–2610 nmol/24 h
Epinephrine	0–20 mcg/24 h	0–109 nmol/24 h

Tests	Conventional Units		SI Units	
Norepinephrine	15–80 mcg/24 h		89–473 nmol/24 h	
CEA, serum				
Nonsmokers	<5.0 ng/mL		<5.0 mcg/L	
Cell counts, adult*				
Erythrocytes				
Male	$4.7–6.1 \times 10^6$/mcL		$4.7–6.1 \times 10^{12}$/L	
Female	$4.2–5.4 \times 10^6$/mcL		$4.2–5.4 \times 10^{12}$/L	
Leukocytes				
Total	$4.8–10.8 \times 10^3$/mcL		$4.8–10.8 \times 10^6$/L	
Differential	Percentage	Absolute	Absolute	
Myelocytes	0	0/mcL	(SI) 0/L	
Neutrophils				
Band	3–5	150–400/ mcL	$150–400 \times 10^6$/L	
Segmented	54–62	3000–5800/ mcL	$3000–5800 \times 10^6$/L	
Lymphocytes	20.5–51.1	$1.2–3.4 \times 10^3$/mcL	$1.2–3.4 \times 10^9$/L	
Monocytes	1.7–9.3	$0.11–0.59 \times 10^3$/mcL	$0.11–0.59 \times 10^9$/L	
Granulocytes	42.2–75.2	$1.4–6.5 \times 10^3$/mcL	$1.4–6.5 \times 10^9$/L	
Eosinophils		$0–0.7 \times 10^3$/mcL	$0–0.7 \times 10^9$/L	
Basophils		$0–0.2 \times 10^3$/mcL	$0–0.2 \times 10^9$/L	
Platelets	$130–400 \times 10^3$/mcL		$130–400 \times 10^9$/L	
Reticulocytes	0.5–1.5% RBCs 24,000–84,000/mcL		0.005–0.015 of RBCs $24–84 \times 10^9$/L	

Tests	Conventional Units	SI Units
Cells, CSF	0–10 lymphocytes/mm^3	0–10 lymphocytes/mm^3
	0 RBC/mm^3	0 RBC/mm^3
Ceruloplasmin, serum	20–60 mg/dL	0.2–0.6 g/L
Chloramphenicol, serum or plasma (Hep or EDTA); trough		
Therapeutic	10–25 mcg/mL	31–77 mcmol/L
Toxic	>25 mcg/mL	>77 mcmol/L
Chloride		
Serum or plasma (Hep)	98–107 mmol/L	98–107 mmol/L
Sweat		
Normal	5–35 mmol/L	5–35 mmol/L
Cystic fibrosis	60–200 mmol/L	60–200 mmol/L
Urine, 24 h (vary greatly with Cl intake)		
Infant	2–10 mmol/24 h	2–10 mmol/24h
Child	15–40 mmol/24 h	15–40 mmol/24h
Adult	110–250 mmol/24 h	110–250 mmol/24 h
CSF	118–132 mmol/L (20 mmol/L higher than serum)	118–132 mmol/L (20 mmol/L higher than serum)
Cholesterol, serum		
Adult		
Desirable	<200 mg/dL	<5.2 mmol/L
Borderline	200–239 mg/dL	5.2–6.2 mmol/L
High-risk	≥240 mg/dL	≥6.2 mmol/L
Cholinesterase, serum*	4.9–11.9 U/mL	4.9–11.9 kU/L
Dibucaine inhibition	79–84%	0.79–0.84

Tests	Conventional Units	SI Units
Fluoride inhibition 58–64%		0.58–0.64
Chorionic gonadotropin, intact*		
Serum or plasma (EDTA)		
Male and nonpregnant female	<5.0 mIU/mL	<5.0 IU/L
Pregnant female	Varies with gestational age	
Urine, qualitative		
Male and nonpregnant female	Negative	Negative
Pregnant female	Positive	Positive
Clonazepam, serum or plasma (Hep or EDTA); trough		
Therapeutic	15–60 ng/mL	48–190 nmol/L
Toxic	>80 ng/mL	>254 nmol/L
Coagulation tests		
Antithrombin III (synthetic substrate)	80–120% of normal	0.8–1.2 of normal
Bleeding time (Duke)	0–6 min	0–6 min
Bleeding time (Ivy)	1–6 min	1–6 min
Bleeding time (template)	2.3–9.5 min	2.3–9.5 min
Clot retraction, qualitative	50–100% in 2 h	0.5–1.0/2 h
Coagulation time (Lee-White)	5–15 min (glass tubes)	5–15 min (glass tubes)

Tests	Conventional Units	SI Units
	19–60 min (siliconized tubes)	19–60 min (siliconized tubes)
Cold hemolysin test (Donath-Landsteiner)	No hemolysis	No hemolysis
Complement components		
Total hemolytic complement activity, plasma (EDTA)	75–160 U/mL	75–160 kU/L
Total complement decay rate (functional), plasma (EDTA)	10–20%	Fraction decay rate: 0.10–0.20
	Deficiency: >50%	>0.50
C1q, serum	14.9–22.1 mg/dL	149–221 mg/L
C1r, serum	2.5–10.0 mg/dL	25–100 mg/L
C1s(C1 esterase), serum	5.0–10.0 mg/dL	50–100 mg/L
C2, serum	1.6–3.6 mg/dL	16–36 mg/L
C3, serum	90–180 mg/dL	0.9–1.8 g/L
C4, serum	10–40 mg/dL	0.1–0.4 g/L
C5, serum	5.5–11.3 mg/dL	55–113 mg/L
C6, serum	17.9–23.9 mg/dL	179–239 mg/L
C7, serum	2.7–7.4 mg/dL	27–74 mg/L
C8, serum	4.9–10.6 mg/dL	49–106 mg/L
C9, serum	3.3–9.5 mg/dL	33–95 mg/L
Coombs test		
Direct	Negative	Negative
Indirect	Negative	Negative

Tests	Conventional Units	SI Units
Copper		
Serum		
Male	70–140 mcg/dL	11–22 mcmol/L
Female	80–155 mcg/dL	13–24 mcmol/L
Urine	3–35 mcg/24 h	0.05–0.55 mcmol/24 h

Corpuscular values of erythrocytes (values are for adults; in children, values vary with age)

Mean corpuscular hemoglobin (MCH)	27–31 pg	0.42–0.48 fmol
Mean corpuscular hemoglobin concentration (MCHC)	33–37 g/dL	330–370 g/L
Mean corpuscular volume (MCV)	Male 80–94 mcm^3	80–94 fL
	Female 81–99 mcm^3	81–99 fL
Cortisol, serum		
Plasma (Hep, EDTA, Ox)		
8 AM	5–23 mcg/dL	138–635 nmol/L
4 PM	3–16 mcg/dL	83–441 nmol/L
10 PM	<50% of 8 AM value	< 0.5 of 8 AM value
Free, urine	<50 mcg/24 h	< 138 mmol/24 h
Creatine kinase (CK), serum*‡		
Male	15–105 U/L (30°C)	0.26–1.79 mckat/L (30°C)
Female	10–80 U/L (30°C)	0.17–1.36 mckat/L (30°C)

(Note: Strenuous exercise or intramuscular injections may elevate transient CK levels.)

Tests	Conventional Units	SI Units
Creatine kinase MB isoenzyme, serum*	0–7 ng/mL	0–7 mcg/L
Creatinine*		
Serum or plasma, adult		
Male	0.7–1.3 mg/dL	62–115 mcmol/L
Female	0.6–1.1 mg/dL	53–97 mcmol/L
Urine		
Male	14–26 mg/kg body weight/24 h	124–230 mcmol/kg body weight/24 h
Female	11–20 mg/kg body weight/24 h	97–177 mcmol/kg body weight/24 h
Creatinine clearance, serum or plasma and urine*		
Male	94–140 mL/min/1.73 m^2	0.91–1.35 mL/s/m^2
Female	72–110 mL/min/1.73 m^2	0.69–1.06 mL/s/m^2
Cryoglobulins, serum	0	0
Cyanide		
Serum		
Nonsmokers	0.004 mg/L	0.15 mcmol/L
Smokers	0.006 mg/L	0.23 mcmol/L
Nitroprusside therapy	0.01–0.06 mg/L	0.38–2.30 mcmol/L
Toxic	>0.1 mg/L	>3.84 mcmol/L
Whole blood (Ox)		
Nonsmokers	0.016 mg/L	0.61 mcmol/L
Smokers	0.041 mg/L	1.57 mcmol/L

Tests	Conventional Units	SI Units
Nitroprusside therapy	0.05–0.5 mg/L	1.92–19.20 mcmol/L
Toxic	>1 mg/L	>38.40 mcmol/L
Cyclic AMP		
Plasma (EDTA)		
Male	4.6–8.6 ng/mL	14–26 nmol/L
Female	4.3–7.6 ng/mL	13–23 nmol/L
Urine, 24 h	0.3–3.6 mg/d	1.0–10.9 mcmol/d or
	or 0.29–2.1 mg/g creatinine	100–723 mcmol/mol creatinine
Cystine or cysteine, urine, qualitative	Negative	Negative
C-Peptide, serum*	0.78–1.89 ng/mL	0.26–0.62 nmol/L
C-Reactive protein, serum	<0.5 mg/dL	<5 mg/L
Cyclosporine, whole blood*§		
Therapeutic, trough	100–200 ng/mL	83–166 nmol/L
Dehydroepiandrosterone (DHEA), serum		
Male	180–1250 ng/dL	6.2–43.3 nmol/L
Female	130–980 ng/dL	4.5–34.0 nmol/L
Dehydroepiandrosterone sulfate (DHEAS) serum or plasma (Hep, EDTA)		
Male	59–452 mcg/mL	1.6–12.2 mcmol/L
Female		
Premenopausal	12–379 mcg/mL	0.8–10.2 mcmol/L

Tests	Conventional Units	SI Units
Postmenopausal	30–260 mcg/mL	0.8–7.1 mcmol/L
Desipramine, serum or plasma (Hep or EDTA); trough (12 h after dose)		
Therapeutic	75–300 ng/mL	281–1125 nmol/L
Toxic	>400 ng/mL	>1500 nmol/L
Diazepam, serum or plasma (Hep or EDTA); trough		
Therapeutic	100–1000 ng/mL	0.35–3.51 mcmol/L
Toxic	>5000 ng/mL	>17.55 mcmol/L
Digitoxin, serum or plasma (Hep or EDTA); 7.8 h after dose		
Therapeutic	20–35 ng/mL	26–46 nmol/L
Toxic	>45 ng/mL	>59 nmol/L
Digoxin, serum or plasma (Hep or EDTA); ≥12 h after dose		
Therapeutic		
CHF	0.8–1.5 ng/mL	1.0–1.9 nmol/L
Arrhythmias	1.5–2.0 ng/mL	1.9–2.6 nmol/L
Toxic		
Adult	>2.5 ng/mL	>3.2 nmol/L
Child	>3.0 ng/mL	>3.8 nmol/L
Disopyramide, serum or plasma (Hep or EDTA); trough		
Therapeutic arrhythmias		
Atrial	2.8–3.2 mcg/mL	8.3–9.4 mcmol/L
Ventricular	3.3–7.5 mcg/mL	9.7–22 mcmol/L
Toxic	>7 mcg/mL	>20.7 mcmol/L
Doxepin, serum or plasma (Hep or EDTA); trough (≥12 h after dose)		
Therapeutic	150–250 ng/mL	537–895 nmol/L
Toxic	>500 ng/mL	>1790 nmol/L

Tests	Conventional Units	SI Units
Estradiol, serum*		
Adult		
Male	10–50 pg/mL	37–184 pmol/L
Female	Varies with menstrual cycle	
Ethanol (alcohol), whole blood (Ox) or serum		
Depression of CNS	>100 mg/dL	>21.7 mmol/L
Fatalities reported	>400 mg/dL	>86.8 mmol/L
Ethosuximide, serum or plasma (Hep or EDTA); trough		
Therapeutic	40–100 mcg/mL	283–708 mcmol/L
Toxic	>150 mcg/mL	>1062 mcmol/L
Euglobin lysis	No lysis in 2 h	No lysis in 2 h
α-Fetoprotein (AFP), serum	<15 ng/mL	<15 mcg/L
Fat, fecal, F, 72 h¶		
Infant, breast-fed	<1 g/d	
Pediatrics (0–6 years)	<2 g/d	
Adult	<7 g/d	
Adult (fat-free diet)	<4 g/d	
Fatty acids, total, serum‖	190–240 mg/dL	7–15 mmol/L
Nonesterified, serum	8–25 mg/dL	0.28–0.89 mmol/L
Ferritin, serum		
Male	20–150 ng/mL	20–250 mcg/L
Female	10–120 ng/mL	10–120 mcg/L

Tests	Conventional Units	SI Units
(Ferritin values of <20 ng/mL (20 mcg/L) have been reported to be generally associated with depleted iron stores.)		
Fibrin degradation products	<10 mcg/mL	<10 mg/L
Fibrinogen, plasma (NaCit)*	200–400 mg/dL	2–4 g/L
Fluoride		
Plasma (Hep)	0.01–0.2 mcg/mL	0.5–10.5 mcmol/L
Urine	0.2–3.2 mcg/mL	10.5–168 mcmol/L
Urine, occupational exposure	<8 mcg/mL	<421 mcmol/L
Folate, Serum RBCs*	3–20 ng/mL	7–45 nmol/L
Erythrocytes	140–628 ng/mL RBC	317–1422 nmol/L RBC
Follicle-stimulating hormone (FSH), serum and plasma (Hep)*		
Male	1.4–15.4 mIU/mL	1.4–15.4 IU/L
Female		
Follicular phase	1–10 mIU/mL	1–10 IU/L
Mid-cycle	6–17 mIU/mL	6–17 IU/L
Luteal phase	1–9 mIU/mL	1–9 IU/L
Postmenopausal	19–100 mIU/mL	19–100 IU/L
Free thyroxine index (FTI), serum*	4.2–13	4.2–13
Gastrin, serum	<100 pg/mL	<100 ng/L

Tests	Conventional Units	SI Units
Gentamicin, serum or plasma (EDTA)		
Therapeutic		
Peak		
Less severe infection	5–8 mcg/mL	10.4–16.7 mcmol
Severe infection	8–10 mcg/mL	16.7–20.9 mcmol/L
Trough		
Less severe infection	<1 mcg/mL	<2.1 mcmol/L
Moderate infection	<2 mcg/mL	<4.2 mcmol/L
Severe infection	<2–4 mcg/mL	<4.2–8.4 mcmol/L
Toxic		
Peak	>10–12 mcg/mL	>21–25 mcmol/L
Trough	>2–4 mcg/mL	>4.2–8.4 mcmol/L
Glucose (fasting)		
Blood	65–95 mg/dL	3.5–5.3 mmol/L
Plasma or serum	74–106 mg/dL	4.1–5.9 mmol/L
Glucose, 2 h postprandial, serum	<120 mg/dL	<6.7 mmol/L
Glucose, urine		
Quantitative	<500 mg/24 h	<2.8 mmol/24 h
Qualitative	Negative	Negative
Glucose, CSF	40–70 mg/dL	2.2–3.9 mmol/L
Glucose-6-phosphate*	12.1 ± 2.1 U/g Hb (SD)	0.78 ± 0.13 mU/mol Hb
Dehydrogenase	351 ± 60.6 U/1012 RBC	0.35 ± 0.06 nU/RBC

Tests	Conventional Units	SI Units
In erythrocytes, whole blood (ACD, EDTA, or Hep)	4.11 ± 0.71 U/mL RBC	4.11 ± 0.71 kU/L RBC
γ-Glutamyltransferase serum		
Males	2–30 U/L (37°C)	0.03–0.51 mckat/L (37°C)
Females	1–24 U/L (37°C)	0.02–0.41 mckat/L (37°C)
Glutethimide, serum		
Therapeutic	2–6 mcg/mL	9–28 mcmol/L
Toxic	>5 mcg/mL	>23 mcmol/L
Glycated hemoglobin (Hemoglobin A1c), whole blood (EDTA)	4.2–5.9%	0.042–0.059
Growth hormone, serum		
Male	<5 ng/mL	<5 mcg/L
Female	<10 ng/mL	<10 mcg/L
Haptoglobin, serum	30–200 mg/dL	0.3–2.0 g/L
HDL-lipid panel†		
Cholesterol, HDL	>40 mg/dL	
Cholesterol, LDL (calculated)		
Optimal	<100 mg/dL	
Near optimal	100–129 mg/dL	
Borderline high	130–159 mg/dL	
High	>160 mg/dL	
Cholesterol, total		
0–1 year	50–120 mg/dL	
1–2 years	70–190 mg/dL	
2–16 years	120–220 mg/dL	

Tests	Conventional Units	SI Units
>16 years	0–199 mg/dL	
desirable	<200 mg/dL	
borderline	200–239 mg/dL	
high	>240 mg/dL	
Triglycerides**		
Desirable	<150 mg/dL	
Borderline high	150–199 mg/dL	
High	>200 mg/dL	
Hematocrit		
Males	42–52%	0.42–0.52
Females	37–47%	0.37–0.47
Newborn	53–65%	0.53–0.65
Children (varies with age)	30–43%	0.30–0.43
Hemoglobin (Hb)		
Males	14.0–18.0 g/dL	2.17–2.79 mmol/L
Females	12.0–16.0 g/dL	1.86–2.48 mmol/L
Newborn	17.0–23.0 g/dL	2.64–3.57 mmol/L
Children (varies with age)	11.2–16.5 g/dL	1.74–2.56 mmol/L
Hemoglobin, fetal	≥1 y old: <2% of total Hb	≥1 y old: <0.02% of total Hb
Hemoglobin, plasma	<3 mg/dL	<0.47 mcmol/L
Hemoglobin and myoglobin, urine, qualitative	Negative	Negative

Tests	Conventional Units	SI Units
Hemoglobin electrophoresis, whole blood (EDTA, Cit, or Hep)		
HbA	>95%	>0.95 Hb fraction
HbA2	1.5–3.7%	0.015–0.037 Hb fraction
HbF	<2%	<0.02 Hb fraction
Homogentisic acid, urine, qualitative	Negative	Negative
β-Hydroxybutyric acid, serum, plasma	0.21–2.81 mg/dL	20–270 mcmol/L
17-Hydroxycorticosteroids, urine		
Males	3–10 mg/24 h	8.3–27.6 mcmol/24 h (as cortisol)
Females	2–8 mg/24 h	5.5–22 mcmol/24 h (as cortisol)
5-Hydroxyindoleacetic acid, urine		
Qualitative	Negative	Negative
Quantitative	2–7 mg/24 h	10.4–36.6 mcmol/24 h
Imipramine, serum or plasma (Hep or EDTA); trough (≥12 h after dose)		
Therapeutic	150–250 ng/mL	536–893 nmol/L
Toxic	>500 ng/mL	>1785 nmol/L
Immunoglobulins, serum		
IgG	700–1600 mg/dL	7–16 g/L
IgA	70–400 mg/dL	0.7–4.0 g/L
IgM	40–230 mg/dL	0.4–2.3 g/L

Tests	Conventional Units	SI Units
IgD	0–8 mg/dL	0–80 mg/L
IgE	3–423 IU/mL	3–423 kIU/L
Immunoglobulin G (IgC), CSF	0.5–6.1 mg/dL	0.5–6.1 g/L
Insulin, plasma (fasting)	2–25 mcU/mL	13–174 pmol/L
Iron, serum*		
Males	65–175 mcg/dL	11.6–31.3 mcmol/L
Females	50–170 mcg/dL	9.0–30.4 mcmol/L
Iron binding capacity, serum, total (TIBC)	250–425 mcg/dL	44.8–71.6 mcmol/L
Iron saturation, serum		
Male	20–50%	0.2–0.5
Female	15–50%	0.15–0.5
17-Ketosteroids, urine		
Males	10–25 mg/24 h	38–87 mcmol/24 h
Females	6–14 mg/24 h (decreases with age)	21–52 mcmol/24 h (decreases with age)
L-Lactate		
Plasma (NaF)		
Venous	4.5–19.8 mg/dL	0.5–2.2 mmol/L
Arterial	4.5–14.4 mg/dL	0.5–1.6 mmol/L
Whole blood (Hep), at bed rest		
Venous	8.1–15.3 mg/dL	0.9–1.7 mmol/L
Arterial	<11.3 mg/dL	<1.3 mmol/L

Tests	Conventional Units	SI Units
Urine, 24 h	496–1982 mg/d	5.5–22 mmol/d
CSF 10–22 mg/dL	1.1–2.4 mmol/L	
Lactate dehydrogenase*		
Total (L→P), 37°C, serum		
Newborn	290–775 U/L	4.9–13.2 mckat/L
Neonate	545–2000 U/L	9.3–34 mckat/L
Infant	180–430 U/L	3.1–7.3 mckat/L
Child	110–295 U/L	1.9–5 mckat/L
Adult	100–190 U/L	1.7–3.2 mckat/L
> 60 years	110–210 U/L	1.9–3.6 mckat/L
Isoenzymes, serum by agarose gel electrophoresis*		
Fraction 1	14–26% of total	0.14–0.26 fraction of total
Fraction 2	29–39% of total	0.29–0.39 fraction of total
Fraction 3	20–26% of total	0.20–0.26 fraction of total
Fraction 4	8–16% of total	0.08–0.16 fraction of total
Fraction 5	6–16% of total	0.06–0.16 fraction of total
Lactate dehydrogenase, CSF*	10% of serum value	0.10 fraction of serum value
LDL-cholesterol (LDL-C), serum or plasma (EDTA)		
Adult desirable	<130 mg/dL	<.2 mmol/L
Borderline	130–159 mg/dL	3.37–4.12 mmol/L
High risk	≥160 mg/dL	≥4.13 mmol/L

Tests	Conventional Units	SI Units
Lead,		
Whole blood (Hep)	<25 mcg/dL	<0.48 mcmol/L
Urine, 24 h	<80 mcg/d	<0.39 mcmol/d
Lecithin-sphingomyelin (L:S) ratio, amniotic fluid	2.0–5.0 indicates probable fetal lung maturity; >3.5 in diabetic patients	2.0–5.0 indicates probable fetal lung maturity; >3.5 in diabetic patients
Lidocaine, serum or plasma (Hep or EDTA); 45 min after bolus dose		
Therapeutic	1.5–6.0 mcg/mL	6.4–26 mcmol/L
Toxic		
CNS, cardiovascular depression	6–8 mcg/mL	26–34.2 mcmol/L
Seizures, obtundation, decreased cardiac output	>8 mcg/mL	>34.2 mcmol/L
Lipase, serum*	23–300 U/L (37°C)	0.39–5.1 mckat/L (37°C)
Lithium, serum or plasma (Hep or EDTA); 12 h after last dose		
Therapeutic	0.6–1.2 mEq/L	0.6–1.2 mmol/L
Toxic	>2 mEq/L	>2 mmol/L
Lorazepam, serum or plasma (Hep or EDTA), therapeutic	50–240 ng/mL	156–746 nmol/L

Tests	Conventional Units	SI Units
Luteinizing hormone (LH), serum or plasma (Hep)*		
Male	1.24–7.8 mIU/mL	1.24–7.8 IU/L
Female		
Follicular phase	1.68–15.0 mIU/mL	1.68–15.0 IU/L
Mid-cycle peak	21.9–56.6 mIU/mL	21.9–56.6 IU/L
Luteal phase	0.61–16.3 mIU/mL	0.61–16.3 IU/L
Postmenopausal	14.2–52.5 mIU/mL	14.2–52.3 IU/L
Magnesium		
Serum	1.3–2.1 mEq/L	0.65–1.07 mmol/L
	1.6–2.6 mg/dL	16–26 mg/L
Urine	6.0–10.0 mEq/24 h	3.0–5.0 mmol/24 h
Mercury		
Whole blood (EDTA)	0.6–59 mcg/L	<0.29 mcmol/L
Urine, 24 h	<20 mcg/d	<0.1 mcmol/d
Toxic	>150 mcg/d	>0.75 mcmol/d
Metanephrines, total, urine	0.1–1.6 mg/24 h	0.5–8.1 mcmol/24 h
Methemoglobin (hemoglobin), whole blood (EDTA, Hep or ACD)	0.06–0.24 g/dL or 0.78 ± 0.37% of total Hb (SD)	9.3–37.2 mcmol/L or mass fraction of total Hb:0.008 ± 0.0037 (SD)
Methotrexate, serum or plasma (Hep or EDTA)		
Therapeutic	Variable	Variable
Toxic		
1–2 weeks after low-dose therapy	≥0.02 mcmol/L	≥0.02 mcmol/L

Tests	Conventional Units	SI Units
Post IV infusion		
24 h	≥5 mcmol/L	≥5 mcmol/L
48 h	≥0.5 mcmol/L	≥0.5 mcmol/L
72 h	≥0.05 mcmol/L	≥0.05 mcmol/L
Myelin basic protein, CSF	<2.5 ng/mL	<2.5 mcg/L
Myoglobin, serum	<85 ng/mL	<85 mcg/L
Nortriptyline, serum or plasma (Hep or EDTA); trough (≥12 h after dose)		
Therapeutic	50–150 ng/mL	190–570 nmol/L
Toxic	>500 ng/mL	>1900 nmol/L
5′-Nucleotidase, serum*	2–17 U/L	0.034–0.29 mckat/L
N-Acetylprocainamide, serum or plasma (Hep or EDTA); trough		
Therapeutic	5–30 mcg/mL	18–108 mcmol/L
Toxic	>40 mcg/mL	>144 mcmol/L
Occult blood, feces, random	Negative (<2 mL blood/150 g stool/d)	Negative (<13.3 mL blood/kg stool/d)
Qualitative, urine, random	Negative	Negative
Osmolality		
Serum	275–295 mOsm/kg serum water	275–295 mmol/kg serum water
Urine	50–1200 mOsm/kg water	50–1200 mmol/kg water
Ratio, urine: serum	1.0–3.0	1.0–3.0
	3.0–4.7 after 12 h fluid restriction	3.0–4.7 after 12 h fluid restriction

Tests	Conventional Units	SI Units
Osmotic fragility of erythrocytes	Begins in 0.45–0.39% NaCl Complete in 0.33–0.30% NaCl	Begins in 77–67 mmol/L NaCl Complete in 56–51 mmol/L NaCl
Oxazepam, serum or plasma (Hep or EDTA), therapeutic	0.2–1.4 mcg/mL	0.70–4.9 mcmol/L
Oxygen, blood		
Capacity	16–24 vol% (varies with hemoglobin)	7.14–10.7 mmol/L (varies with hemoglobin)
Content		
Arterial	15–23 vol%	6.69–10.3 mmol/L
Venous	10–16 vol%	4.46–7.14 mmol/L
Saturation		
Arterial and capillary	95–98% of capacity	0.95–0.98 of capacity
Venous	60–85% of capacity	0.60–0.85 of capacity
Tension		
pO_2 arterial and capillary	83–108 mmHg	11.1–14.4 kPa
Venous	35–45 mmHg	4.6–6.0 kPa
P50, blood	25–29 mmHg (adjusted to pH 7.4)	3.33–3.86 kPa
Partial thromboplastin time activated (APTT)	<35 sec	<35 sec

Tests	Conventional Units	SI Units
Pentobarbital, serum or plasma (Hep or EDTA); trough		
Therapeutic		
Hypnotic	1–5 mcg/mL	4–22 mcmol/L
Therapeutic coma	20–50 mcg/mL	88–221 mcmol/L
Toxic	>10 mcg/mL	>44 mcmol/L
pH		
Blood, arterial	7.35–7.45	7.35–7.45
Urine	4.6–8.0 (depends on diet)	Same
Phenacetin, plasma (EDTA)		
Therapeutic	1–30 mcg/mL	6–167 mcmol/L
Toxic	50–250 mcg/mL	279–1395 mcmol/L
Phenobarbital, serum or plasma (Hep or EDTA); trough		
Therapeutic	15–40 mcg/mL	65–172 mcmol/L
Toxic		
Slowness, ataxia, nystagmus	35–80 mcg/mL	151–345 mcmol/L
Coma with reflexes	65–117 mcg/mL	280–504 mcmol/L
Coma without reflexes	>100 mcg/mL	>430 mcmol/L
Phenolsulfon- phthalein (PSP) excretion, urine	28–51% in 15 min	0.28–0.51 in 15 min
	13–24% in 30 min	0.13–0.24 in 30 min
	9–17% in 60 min	0.09–0.17 in 60 min

Tests	Conventional Units	SI Units
	3–10% in 2 h (After injection of 1 mL PSP intravenously)	0.03–0.10 in 2 h (After injection of 1 mL PSP intravenously)
Phenylalanine, serum	0.8–1.8 mg/dL	48–109 mcmol/L
Phenytoin, serum or plasma (Hep or EDTA); trough		
Therapeutic	10–20 mcg/mL	40–79 mcmol/L
Toxic	>20 mcg/mL	>79 mcmol/L
Phosphatase, acid, prostatic, serum radioimmunoassay*	<3.0 ng/mL	<3.0 mcg/L
Phosphatase, alkaline, total, serum*	38–126 U/L (37°C)	0.65–2.14 mckat/L
Phosphate, inorganic, serum		
Adults	2.7–4.5 mg/dL	0.87–1.45 mmol/L
Children	4.5–5.5 mg/dL	1.45–1.78 mmol/L
Phosphatidylglycerol, amniotic fluid		
Fetal lung immaturity	absent	absent
Fetal lung maturity	present	present
Phospholipids, serum	125–275 mg/dL	1.25–2.75 g/L
Phosphorus, urine	0.4–1.3 g/24 h	12.9–42 mmol/24 h
Porphobilinogen, urine		
Qualitative	Negative	Negative
Quantitative	<2.0 mg/24 h	<9 mcmol/24 h

Tests	Conventional Units	SI Units
Porphyrins, urine		
Coproporphyrin	34–230 mcg/24 h	52–351 nmol/24 h
Uroporphyrin	27–52 mcg/24 h	32–63 nmol/24 h
Potassium, plasma (Hep)		
Males	3.5–4.5 mEq/L	3.5–4.5 mmol/L
Females	3.4–4.4 mEq/L	3.4–4.4 mmol/L
Potassium		
Serum		
Premature		
Cord	5.0–10.2 mEq/L	5.0–10.2 mmol/L
48 h	3.0–6.0 mEq/L	3.0–6.0 mmol/L
Newborn, cord	5.6–12.0 mEq/L	5.6–12.0 mmol/L
Newborn	3.7–5.9 mEq/L	3.7–5.9 mmol/L
Infant	4.1–5.3 mEq/L	4.1–5.3 mmol/L
Child	3.4–4.7 mEq/L	3.4–4.7 mmol/L
Adult	3.5–5.1 mEq/L	3.5–5.1 mmol/L
Urine, 24 h (varies with diet)	25–125 mEq/d	25–125 mmol/d
CSF	70% of plasma level or 2.5–3.2 mEq/L; rises with plasma hyperosmolality	0.70 of plasma level or 2.5–3.2 mmol/L; rises with plasma hyperosmolality
Prealbumin (transthyretin), serum	10–40 mg/dL	100–400 mg/L
Primidone, serum or plasma (Hep or EDTA); trough		
Therapeutic	5–12 mcg/mL	23–55 mcmol/L
Toxic	>15 mcg/mL	>69 mcmol/L

Tests	Conventional Units	SI Units
Procainamide, serum or plasma (Hep or EDTA); trough		
Therapeutic	4–10 mcg/mL	17–42 mcmol/L
Toxic (also consider effect of metabolite, i.e., NAPA)	>10–12 mcg/mL	>42–51 mcmol/L
Progesterone, serum*		
Adult		
Male	13–97 ng/dL	0.4–3.1 nmol/L
Female		
Follicular phase	15–70 ng/dL	0.5–2.2 nmol/L
Luteal phase	200–2500 ng/dL	6.4–79.5 nmol/L
Pregnancy	Varies with gestational week	
Prolactin, serum*		
Males	2.5–15.0 ng/mL	2.5–15.0 mcg/L
Females	2.5–19.0 ng/mL	2.5–19.0 mcg/L
Propoxyphene, plasma (EDTA)		
Therapeutic	0.1–0.4 mcg/mL	0.3–1.2 mcmol/L
Toxic	>0.5 mcg/mL	>1.5 mcmol/L
Propranolol, serum or plasma (Hep or EDTA); trough		
Therapeutic	50–100 ng/mL	193–386 nmol/L
Prostate-specific antigen (PSA), serum*		
Male	<4.0 ng/mL	<4.0 mcg/L
Protein, serum*		
Total	6.4–8.3 g/dL	64–83 g/L
Albumin	3.9–5.1 g/dL	39–51 g/L
Globulin		
α_1	0.2–0.4 g/dL	2–4 g/L
α_2	0.4–0.8 g/dL	4–8 g/L

Tests	Conventional Units	SI Units
β	0.5–1.0 g/dL	5–10 g/L
γ	0.6–1.3 g/dL	6–13 g/L
Urine		
Qualitative	Negative	Negative
Quantitative	50–80 mg/24 h (at rest)	Same
CSF, total	8–32 mg/dL	80–320 mg/dL
Prothrombin consumption	>20 sec	>20 sec
Prothrombin time-international normalized ratio		
INR: birth–6 months	1.0–1.6	
INR: 6 months–adult	0.9–1.2	
Protoporphyrin, total, WB	<60 mcg/dL	<600 mcg/L
Pyruvate, blood	0.3–0.9 mg/dL	34–103 mcmol/L
Quinidine, serum or plasma (Hep or EDTA); trough		
Therapeutic	2–5 mcg/mL	6–15 mcmol/L
Toxic	>6 mcg/mL	>18 mcmol/L
Salicylates, serum or plasma (Hep or EDTA); trough		
Therapeutic	150–300 mcg/mL	1.09–2.17 mmol/L
Toxic	>500 mcg/mL	>3.62 mmol/L
Sedimentation rate, erythrocyte[††]		
Westergren		
Male: 0–50 years	0–15 mm/h	
Male: >50 years	0–20 mm/h	
Female: 0–50 years	0–20 mm/h	

Tests	Conventional Units	SI Units
Female: >50 years	0–30 mm/h	
Wintrobe		
Males	<10 mm/h	
Females	<20 mm/h	
Critical value	>75 mm/h	
Sodium		
Serum or plasma (Hep)		
Premature		
Cord	116–140 mEq/L	116–140 mmol/L
48 h	128–148 mEq/L	128–148 mmol/L
Newborn, cord	126–166 mEq/L	126–166 mmol/L
Newborn	133–146 mEq/L	133–146 mmol/L
Infant	139–146 mEq/L	139–146 mmol/L
Child	138–145 mEq/L	138–145 mmol/L
Adult	136–145 mEq/L	136–145 mmol/L
Urine, 24 h	40–220 mEq/d (diet dependent)	40–220 mmol/d (diet dependent)
Sweat		
Normal	10–40 mEq/L	10–40 mmol/L
Cystic fibrosis	70–190 mEq/L	70–190 mmol/L
Specific gravity, urine	1.002–1.030	1.002–1.030
Testosterone, serum*		
Male	280–1100 ng/dL	0.52–38.17 nmol/L
Female	15–70 ng/dL	0.52–2.43 nmol/L
Pregnancy	3–4 × normal	3–4 × normal
Postmenopausal	8–35 ng/dL	0.28–1.22 nmol/L

Tests	Conventional Units	SI Units
Theophylline, serum or plasma (Hep or EDTA)		
Therapeutic		
Bronchodilator	8–20 mcg/mL	44–111 mcmol/L
Prem. apnea	6–13 mcg/mL	33–72 mcmol/L
Toxic	>20 mcg/mL	>110 mcmol/L
Thiocyanate		
Serum or plasma (EDTA)		
Nonsmoker	1–4 mcg/mL	17–69 mcmol/L
Smoker	3–12 mcg/mL	52–206 mcmol/L
Therapeutic after nitroprusside infusion	6–29 mcg/mL	103–499 mcmol/L
Urine		
Nonsmoker	1–4 mg/d	17–69 mcmol/d
Smoker	7–17 mg/d	120–292 mcmol/d
Thiopental, serum or plasma (Hep or EDTA); trough		
Hypnotic	1.0–5.0 mcg/mL	4.1–20.7 mcmol/L
Coma	30–100 mcg/mL	124–413 mcmol/L
Anesthesia	7–130 mcg/mL	29–536 mcmol/L
Toxic concentration	>10 mcg/mL	>41 mcmol/L
Thyroid-stimulating hormone (TSH), serum*	0.4–4.2 mcU/mL	0.4–4.2 mU/L
Thyroxine (T_4) serum	5–12 mcg/dL (varies with age, higher in children and pregnant women)	65–155 nmol/L (varies with age, higher in children and pregnant women)

Tests	Conventional Units	SI Units
Thyroxine, free, serum*	0.8–2.7 ng/dL	10.3–35 pmol/L
Thyroxine binding globulin (TBG), serum	1.2–3.0 mg/dL	12–30 mg/L
Tobramycin, serum or plasma (Hep or EDTA)		
Therapeutic		
Peak		
Less severe infection	5–8 mcg/mL	11–17 mcmol/L
Severe infection	8–10 mcg/mL	17–21 mcmol/L
Trough		
Less severe infection	<1 mcg/mL	<2 mcmol/L
Moderate infection	<2 mcg/mL	<4 mcmol/L
Severe infection	<2–4 mcg/mL	<4–9 mcmol/L
Toxic		
Peak	>10–12 mcg/mL	>21–26 mcmol/L
Trough	>2–4 mcg/mL	>4–9 mcmol/L
Transferrin, serum		
Newborn	130–275 mg/dL	1.30–2.75 g/L
Adult	212–360 mg/dL	2.12–3.60 g/L
>60 years	190–375 mg/dL	1.9–3.75 g/L
Triglycerides, serum, fasting		
Desirable	<250 mg/dL	<2.83 mmol/L
Borderline high	250–500 mg/dL	2.83–5.67 mmol/L
Hypertrigly-ceridemia	>500 mg/dL	>5.65 mmol/L

Tests	Conventional Units	SI Units
Triiodothyronine, total (T_3) serum*	100–200 ng/dL	1.54-3.8 nmol/L
Troponin-I, cardiac, serum*	undetectable	undetectable
Troponin-T, cardiac, serum	undetectable	undetectable
Urea nitrogen, serum	6–20 mg/dL	2.1–7.1 mmol urea/L
Urea nitrogen: creatinine ratio, serum	12:1 to 20:1	48–80 urea: creatinine mole ratio
Uric acid*		
Serum, enzymatic		
Male	4.5–8.0 mg/dL	0.27–0.47 mmol/L
Female	2.5–6.2 mg/dL	0.15–0.37 mmol/L
Child	2.0–5.5 mg/dL	0.12–0.32 mmol/L
Urine	250–750 mg/ 24 h (with normal diet)	1.48–4.43 mmol/24 h (with normal diet)
Urobilinogen, urine	0.1–0.8 Ehrlich unit/2 h	0.1-0.8 Eu/2h
	0.5–4.0 Eu/d	0.5-4.0 Eu/d
Valproic acid, serum or plasma (Hep or EDTA); trough		
Therapeutic	50–100 mcg/mL	347–693 mcmol/L
Toxic	>100 mcg/mL	>693 mcmol/L

Tests	Conventional Units	SI Units
Vancomycin, serum or plasma (Hep or EDTA)		
Therapeutic		
Peak	20–40 mcg/mL	14–28 mcmol/L
Trough	5–10 mcg/mL	3–7 mcmol/L
Toxic	>80–100 mcg/mL	>55–69 mcmol/L
Vanillylmandelic acid (VMA), urine (4-hydroxy-3-methoxymandelic acid)	1.4–6.5 mg/24 h	7–33 mcmol/d
Viscosity, serum	1.00–1.24 cP	1.00–1.24 cP
Vitamin A, serum	30–80 mcg/dL	1.05–2.8 mcmol/L
Vitamin B12, serum	110–800 pg/mL	81–590 pmol/L
Vitamin E, serum		
Normal	5–18 mcg/mL	12–42 mcmol/L
Therapeutic	30–50 mcg/mL	69.6–116 mcmol/L
Zinc, serum	70–120 mcg/dL	10.7–18.4 mcmol/L

Notes on INR: INR = (Patient PT / Normal PT) × ISI, where ISI is the international sensitivity index, a value provided by the reagent manufacturer. Target therapeutic range is 2.0–3.0 (source: http://pediatrics.aappublications.org/cgi/content/full/112/5/e386). The American College of Chest Physicians has recommended a therapeutic INR range for adults of 2.0–3.0, except in patients with mechanical cardiac valves who should have an INR of 2.5–3.5, a target INR range of 2.6–3.8 for children with heart disease, and a slightly lower range of 2.1–3.3 for treating children with established venous thrombosis. Clinicians at Toronto's Hospital for Sick Children used an INR range of 2.0–3.0 initially but later found that a lower target of 1.3–1.8 was as effective and resulted in no bleeding complications. http://www.healthsystem.virginia.edu/internet/pediatrics/pharma-news/jan95.pdf. The recommended therapeutic target for the treatment and prevention of venous thromboembolisms and pulmonary embolisms in an INR of 2.5 with a range between 2.0–3.0, and children with mechanical prosthetic heart valves have a recommended therapeutic INR range of 3.0 INR range between 2.5–3.5. Evaluate at that time (source: http://www.warfarinfo.com/pediatrics.htm).

*Test values dependent on laboratory methods used.

†Source: https://labs-sec.uhs-sa.com/clinical_ext/dols/soprefrange.asp.

‡Test values dependent on patient's race.

§Actual therapeutic range should be adjusted for individual patient.

¶Reference values vary from laboratory to laboratory, but are generally found within the range of 5–7 g/d. It should be noted that children, especially infants, cannot ingest the 100 g/d of fat that is suggested for the test. Therefore, a fat retention coefficient is determined by measuring the difference between ingested fat and fecal fat, and expressing that difference as a percentage. The figure, called the fat retention coefficient, is 95% or greater in healthy children and adults. A low value indicates steatorrhea. Source: http://www.labcorp.com/datasets/labcorp/html/chapter/mono/sc008000.htm.

∥"Fatty acids" include a mixture of different aliphatic acids of varying molecular weight; a mean molecular weight of 284 daltons has been assumed.

**If the triglyceride value is >400 mg/dL, the LDL calculation is invalid. Source: http://webserver01.bjc.org/slch/pro/Professional.htm? and http://webserver01.bjc.org/labtestguide/Lab%20Test%20Guidebook/slchlabsiteoneline.htm.

#http://www.labcorp.com/datasets/labcorp/html/chapter/mono/he005000.htm; http://www.utmb.edu/lsg/LabSurvivalGuide/hem/Sedimentation_Rate.htm.

Diagnostic Tests and Procedures

Name/ Synonyms	Indication(s)	Description/ Specimen
Abdominal aorta sonogram; ultrasonography	To detect and measure suspected abdominal aortic aneurysm	Ultrasound waves sent into the body with a small transducer; sound waves are transformed into a visual display on the monitor
Acid-fast bacilli (AFB)	To identify mycobacteria in sputum specimens	Sputum that is sent for Gram stain
Adrenocortico-tropic hormone (ACTH); corticotropin	To evaluate adrenal cortical dysfunction	Blood sample
Alanine aminotransferase (ALT); formerly serum glutamic-pyruvic transaminase (SGPT)	To monitor liver damage	Blood sample
Aldosterone	To diagnose primary and secondary aldosteronism	Blood and urine samples
Alkaline phosphatase (ALP)	To measure serum levels of alkaline phosphatase, an enzyme that is	Blood sample

Name/ Synonyms	Indication(s)	Description/ Specimen
	increased in bone growth, liver disease, biliary obstruction, osteogenic sarcoma, or breast or prostate cancer with metastases to the bone	
Allergen-specific IgE antibody; radioallergosorbent test (RAST test); allergy screen	To test for allergies to allergens	Blood sample
Alpha-fetoprotein (AFP)	To test for neural tube defects in the fetus such as spina bifida and anencephaly	Blood sample
Ambulatory electrocardiography; ambulatory monitoring; event monitoring; Holter monitoring	To monitor electrical activity of the heart and to detect arrhythmias which occur sporadically	Electrodes are applied to the skin, monitor and case are positioned, and the recorder is turned on
Ammonia	To assess for accumulation of ammonia in the bloodstream	Blood sample

Name/ Synonyms	Indication(s)	Description/ Specimen
Amylase	To assess for pancreatitis, diabetic ketoacidosis, cirrhosis, hepatitis, cholelithiasis, hyperthyroidism, or other conditions	Blood or urine sample
Angiotensin-converting enzyme (ACE); serum angiotensin-converting enzyme	To assess for diabetic retinopathy, Gaucher disease, hyperthyroidism, liver disease, or sarcoidosis	Blood sample
Anion gap	To determine causes of metabolic acidosis including those associated with renal failure, diabetic ketoacidosis, or lactic acidosis	Blood sample
Anti-DNA antibody test	Detects presence of antibodies to native or double-stranded DNA, indicating some type of autoimmune disease	Blood sample

Name/ Synonyms	Indication(s)	Description/ Specimen
Antinuclear antibody test (ANA)	Used to rule out systemic lupus erythematosus, endocarditis, cirrhosis, connective tissue diseases, and chronic autoimmune hepatitis	Blood sample
Arterial blood gas (ABG) analysis; blood gases	For information regarding the acid-base status of the patient	Blood sample
Arteriography of the lower extremities; lower extremity angiography	Visualization of blood vessels	Contrast dye is injected through a catheter into an artery; radiographic films are then taken of the artery
Arthrocentesis; synovial fluid analysis	To diagnose arthritis, to investigate joint effusion, or to remove excess fluid from the joint	Synovial fluid sample
Arthrogram	To assess for joint damage and/or cartilage tears	Injection of radiopaque dye or air into the joint; radiographs are taken as the joint is manipulated

Name/ Synonyms	Indication(s)	Description/ Specimen
Arthroscopy	To directly visualize joint structures and to perform biopsy and simple repairs	The arthroscope is inserted into the joint spaces; the joint is manipulated as it is visualized
Aspartate aminotransferase (AST); formerly serum glutamic oxaloacetic transaminase (SGOT)	To assess for heart muscle damage as in myocardial infarction; to assess for liver damage	Blood sample
Barium enema; large bowel study; lower GI series	Fluoroscopic examination of the large intestines for lower abdominal pain, changes in bowel habits, stools containing blood or mucus, visualizing polyps, diverticula or tumors	The entire intestine is filled from the rectum to the ileocecal valve; the area is observed on a fluoroscopic screen with films taken periodically
Barium swallow; esophageal radiography; esophagography	To evaluate dysphagia or regurgitation, hiatal hernia, diverticula, achalasia, esophagitis, polyps, and/or strictures	Patient swallows a thick barium mixture for fluoroscopic exam of the pharynx and esophagus; part of upper GI series

Name/ Synonyms	Indication(s)	Description/ Specimen
Bilirubin, direct (conjugated); indirect bilirubin indirect (unconjugated); total bilirubin	To assess for choledocholithiasis, cirrhosis, hepatitis, myocardial infarction, pernicious anemia, and/or septicemia	Blood sample
Bleeding time; aspirin tolerance test; Duke bleeding time; ivy bleeding time; modified ivy; template bleeding time	To screen for disorders involving platelet function and vascular defects that interfere with clotting	A standard skin incision is made usually just below the crease of the elbow; blood drops are blotted every 30 seconds; time is stopped when bleeding ceases
Blood alcohol; ethanol; ethyl alcohol (ETOH)	To screen for alcohol ingestion	Blood sample
Blood culture and sensitivity	To screen for bacteria in the blood	Blood sample
Blood smear; peripheral blood smear; red blood cell smear (RBC smear)	Examines cells in terms of size, shape, color, and structure	Blood sample
Blood typing; ABO typing; ABO red cell groups; blood groups; Rh typing; type and	To determine an individual's blood type, Rh factors in the blood, and	Blood sample

Name/ Synonyms	Indication(s)	Description/ Specimen
crossmatch (T&C); type and screen	compatibility in donor blood	
Bone marrow biopsy; bone marrow aspiration	To screen for cancer, depressed hematopoiesis, granuloma, infection, iron-deficiency anemia, leukemia, multiple myeloma, polycythemia vera, or thalassemia	A large-bore needle is advanced through the subcutaneous tissue cortex of bone to aspirate a sample of bone marrow
Bone scan	To detect metastatic cancer of the bone and monitor the progression of degenerative bone disorders; to detect fractures in patients with continued pain when x-rays have been negative	A radionuclide is injected intravenously; scintillation camera takes radioactivity reading from the body and transforms them into two-dimensional pictures of the skeleton
Brain scan (cerebral blood flow)	To assess for brain abscess, tumors, contusions, hematomas or cerebrovascular	A radionuclide is injected intravenously; scintillation camera takes radioactivity reading from the head and

Name/ Synonyms	Indication(s)	Description/ Specimen
	accidents (CVAs); interruption of the blood-brain barrier	transforms them into two-dimensional pictures of the brain
Breast biopsy	To assess for malignancy	Needle biopsy: a sample of tissue is aspirated into a syringe for examination Open biopsy: an excision is made over the breast mass, which is excised in its entirety for testing
Bronchoscopy	To visualize abnormalities found on radiography, obtain sputum specimens, remove foreign bodies, conduct endobronchial radiation, or obliterate neoplastic obstruction	The bronchoscope is introduced through the mouth or nose; the anatomy of the trachea and bronchi are inspected
CA15-3, CA19-9, CA-125, tumor markers/ antigens	To assess for the presence of cancer	Blood sample

Name/ Synonyms	Indication(s)	Description/ Specimen
Calcitonin; thyrocalcitonin	To assess for hypercalcemia	Blood sample
Calcium	To assess calcium level	Blood or urine sample
Candida antibody test	To assess for Candida infection	Blood sample
Carboxyhemo- globin; carbon monoxide (CO)	To assess for carbon monoxide poisoning	Blood sample
Carcinoem- bryonic antigen (CEA)	To assess carcinoembryonic antigen levels for malignancy	Blood sample
Cardiac catheterization; angiocardiogra- phy, coronary angiography; coronary arteriography; heart catheterization	Visualization of the blood vessels to assess for heart size, structure, movement, wall thickness, blood flow, valve motion, and/or coronary vasculature	A catheter is inserted through an artery into the correct position and dye is inserted; radiographic films are taken of the artery
Carotid duplex scanning; carotid phonoangiogra- phy (CPA)	To assess for plaque, stenosis, or partial occlusion of arteries	A transducer is placed on the skin; sound waves are transformed into a visual display on the monitor

Name/ Synonyms	Indication(s)	Description/ Specimen
Cerebral angiography; cerebral arteriography	To detect cerebrovascular abnormalities such as aneurysm or arteriovenous malformation, to study vascular displacement, or to evaluate postoperative status of blood vessels	A catheter is inserted through an artery into the correct position and dye is inserted; radiographic films are taken of the artery
Cerebrospinal fluid (CSF) analysis; cisternal puncture; lumbar puncture (LP); spinal tap; ventricular puncture	To assist in the diagnosis of a wide variety of central nervous system diseases, including infectious diseases	A sample of cerebrospinal fluid is collected using a spinal needle
Chemistry profile	To assess multiple organ systems to determine overall health and wellness	May include alanine aminotransferase (ALT); alkaline phosphatase (ALP); aspartate aminotransferase (AST); bilirubin; calcium; carbon dioxide; chloride; cholesterol; creatinine kinase (CK); creatinine; gamma-glutamyl

Name/ Synonyms	Indication(s)	Description/ Specimen
		transferase (GGT); glucose; lactic dehydrogenase (LDH); phosphorus; potassium; protein; sodium; triglyc- erides; urea nitrogen; and uric acid tests
Chest x-ray (CXR); chest radiography	To identify abnormalities of the lungs and other structures of the thorax including heart, ribs, and diaphragm	X-ray of the chest
Chlamydia	To assess for Chlamydia trachomatis or trachoma	Titer: Blood sample Eye culture: Swab of inner canthus or lower conjunctiva Cervical culture: Swab of the cervix
Chloride	To evaluate the chloride level in the blood or kidneys	Blood or urine sample
Cholecystogra- phy; gallbladder radiography; gallbladder series; oral cholecystogram	To assess for gallbladder disease	After ingestion of a contrast medium, films are taken of the right upper quadrant in three positions

Name/ Synonyms	Indication(s)	Description/ Specimen
Cholesterol	To evaluate LDL and HDL and risk potential for atherosclerosis and heart disease	Blood sample
Clostridium difficile (*C. difficile*) toxin assay; clostridial toxin assay	To evaluate for pseudomembranous colitis	Stool specimen
Coagulation factor assay; factor assay; clotting factors	To assess for congential or acquired deficiency of blood clotting factor	Blood sample
Coagulation studies	To evaluate coagulation disorders	Include antithrombin III; bleeding time; clot retraction; coagulation factors; D-dimer; euglobulin lysis time; fibrin degradation; fibrinogen; partial thromboplastin time; plasminogen; protein C; protein S; prothrombin time; and thrombin clotting time tests

Name/ Synonyms	Indication(s)	Description/ Specimen
Colonoscopy	To assess lower GI bleeding, change in bowel habits, high risk for colon cancer due to polyps, or ulcerative colitis or history	Direct visualization of the large intestine through the use of a flexible fiberoptic endoscope
Colposcopy; endometrial biopsy	To identify the area of cellular dysplasia	Direct visualization of the cervix and vagina with a colposcope with magnifying lens and light
Complete blood cell count with differential (CBC with diff)	To evaluate red blood counts, white blood counts, and platelets	Includes blood smear; hematocrit; hemoglobin, platelets; RBC count; RBC indices (MCV, MCH, MCHC); WBC count; and differential
Computed tomography (CT) of the abdomen; CT scan of the abdomen; computerized axial tomography (CAT) of the abdomen	To diagnose pathologic conditions of the abdominal organs including inflammation, cysts, tumors of the liver, gallbladder, pancreas, spleen, kidneys, and pelvic organs	Contrast dye is given by IV injection; films are taken in the body scanner

Name/ Synonyms	Indication(s)	Description/ Specimen
Computed tomography (CT) of the brain; CT scan of the head; computerized axial tomography (CAT) of the head	To diagnose pathologic conditions such as neoplasms, cerebral infarctions, aneurysm, and intracranial hemorrhage	Contrast dye is given by IV injection; films are taken in the body scanner
Computed tomography (CT) of the chest; CT scan of the chest; computerized axial tomography (CAT) of the chest	To diagnose pathologic conditions, including inflammation, cysts, and tumors of the lungs, esophagus, and lymph nodes	Contrast dye is given by IV injection; films are taken in the body scanner
Coombs test, direct; direct antiglobulin test; red blood cell (RBC) antibody screen	To assess if antibodies are attached to the red blood cells, indicating infectious mononucleosis or systemic lupus erythematosus; to detect red blood cell sensitization to drugs or blood transfusions	Blood sample
Coombs test, indirect;	To detect unexpected circulating	Blood sample

Name/ Synonyms	Indication(s)	Description/ Specimen
antibody screening test	antibodies that may react against transfused red blood cells, other than those of the ABO groups	
Cortisol	To assess for normal function of the anterior pituitary gland	Blood or urine sample
C-reactive protein test (CRP)	To assess for inflammatory process	Blood sample
Creatine kinase (CK) and isoenzymes; formerly creatine phosphokinase (CPK)	To assess for myocardial infarction	Blood sample
Creatinine; creatinine clearance	To evaluate renal function	Blood and/or urine sample
Cystometry; cystometro-graphy (CMG)	To evaluate detrusor instability and cause of bladder dysfunction	Instillation of fluid and/or air into the bladder, assessment of neurologic and muscular responses to this filling, and assessment of patient's voiding for abnormalities

Name/ Synonyms	Indication(s)	Description/ Specimen
Cystourethro-graphy	To evaluate chronic urinary tract infections (UTIs)	Instillation of contrast medium into the bladder through a urethral catheter; x-ray films are taken as the bladder fills and as the patient voids
Cystourethro-scopy; cystoscopy; urethroscopy	Calculi removal, diagnosis; other therapeutic procedures other than calculi removal: obstruction, urothelial carcinoma, filling defects, unilateral gross hematuria, malignant cytology, survei-llance, passage of ureteral catheter for obstruction of fistula, foreign body, resection/fulguration of selected tumors, and dilation/incision of strictures	Passing of cystoscope into the bladder to visualize the urinary tract
Disseminated intravascular coagulation screening (DIC screening)	To assess when both clotting and bleeding occur at abnormally high levels	See coagulation studies

Name/ Synonyms	Indication(s)	Description/ Specimen
Doppler studies; Doppler ultrasonography	To evaluate blood flow in the major veins and arteries of the legs, arms, and neck	Ultrasound waves are sent into the body with a small transducer pressed against the skin
Echocardiography; echo; heart sonogram	To assess heart chambers, valves, blood flow or muscle	Ultrasound waves are sent into the body with a small transducer pressed against the skin
Electrocardiography, electrocardiogram (ECG, EKG)	To record the electrical current generated by the heart	Monitoring electrodes are placed on the body
Electroencephalography (EEG)	To record the electrical activity of the brain	Monitoring electrodes are placed on the scalp
Electromyography, electromyelography (EMG)	To record the electrical activity in the skeletal muscle groups	Insertion of needle electrodes into the muscle
Electroneurography, electromyoneurography (ENG)	To assess for peripheral nerve disease or injury	Electrodes over a nerve initiate electrical impulse at the proximal site; time is recorded for the impulse to reach a distal site on the same nerve

Name/ Synonyms	Indication(s)	Description/ Specimen
Endoscopic retrograde cholangiopancreatography (ERCP)	To assess for obstructive jaundice, cancer, calculi, or stenosis	Radiographic viewing of the pancreatic ducts and hepatobiliary tree through an endoscope
Erythrocyte sedimentation rate (ESR), sedimentation rate (sed rate); Westergren; Wintrobe	To assess for inflammatory and necrotic conditions	Blood sample
Esophageal manometry; acid reflux test; Bernstein test; esophageal function studies	To assess the esophagus for normal contractile activity	Manometric catheter is placed at various levels in the esophagus; baseline pressure measurements are taken as the patient swallows
Esophagogastro-duodenoscopy (EGD); esophagoscopy; gastroscopy; upper gastrointestinal (GI) endoscopy	To assess the esophagus, stomach, and upper duodenum via direct visualization	The endoscope is inserted through the mouth to inspect anatomy, remove tissue specimen, and/or remove foreign bodies
Estradiol receptor and progesterone	To assess whether breast cancer	Specimen of breast tissue is

Name/ Synonyms	Indication(s)	Description/ Specimen
receptor (ER/PR) in breast cancer; ER/PR assay	tissue would respond to treatment to reduce the hormone level	removed by excision or needle biopsy
Estrogen; estrogen total; estrogen fractions; estradiol; estriol	To evaluate adrenal cortex, ovaries, and testes function	Blood sample
Evoked potential studies (EP studies); evoked responses; auditory brainstem-evoked potentials; somatosensory evoked potentials; visual evoked potentials	To diagnose lesions of the nervous system by evaluating integrity of the visual, somatosensory, and auditory nerve pathways	Electrodes are placed in appropriate positions and recordings measured
Exercise electrocardio-graphy (exercise ECG); graded exercise tolerance test; stress testing; treadmill test	Measures the efficiency of the heart during physical activity	Electrocardiography and blood pressure monitoring while the patient walks a treadmill; pharmacological stress through adenosine, dipyridamole and dobutamine rather than exercise

Name/ Synonyms	Indication(s)	Description/ Specimen
Fecal fat	To evaluate for steatorrhea in Crohn disease, cystic fibrosis, or Whipple disease	Stool samples for three days
Ferritin	To evaluate the size of iron storage compartments; to diagnose anemia	Blood sample
Folic acid; folate	To diagnose macrocytic anemia	Blood sample
Follicle-stimulating hormone (FSH)	To diagnose hypogonadism, infertility, menstrual disorders, or precocious puberty	Blood sample
Free erythrocyte protoporphyrin (FEP)	To detect iron-deficiency anemia	Blood sample
Gallbladder scan; hepatobiliary imaging; HIDA scan	To assess for cholecystitis or obstruction of the cystic duct	Injection of a radionuclide compound; visualization of the biliary system using a scintillation camera
Gallium scan; body scan	To detect primary neoplasms, metastatic lesions,	Injection of radioactive gallium citrate; a scintillation camera is used to

Name/ Synonyms	Indication(s)	Description/ Specimen
	and inflammatory processes	scan the entire body
Gamma-glutamyl transferase (GGT); gamma-glutamyl transpeptidase (GGTP)	To assist in the diagnosis of liver problems	Blood sample
Glucose tolerance test (GTT); oral glucose tolerance test (OGTT)	To assess the rate at which glucose is removed from the bloodstream	Blood and urine sample
Glucose, postprandial; 2-hour postprandial blood sugar (2-hour PPBS); 2-hour p.c. glucose	To assess response of the body to ingestion of a meal with a standard amount of carbohydrates; to assess for effectiveness of insulin therapy	Blood sample
Glucose; blood sugar; fasting blood sugar (FBS); fasting plasma glucose (FPG)	To assess for problems with glucose metabolism	Blood sample

Name/ Synonyms	Indication(s)	Description/ Specimen
Glycosylated hemoglobin (G-Hb); glycated Hgb; glyco-hemoglobin; hemoglobin A_{1c} (HbA_{1c}, $HgbA_{1c}$)	To determine the average blood glucose level for the previous two to three months	Blood sample
Gonorrhea culture	To test for *Neisseria gonorrhoeae*	Endocervical culture: swab of cervical mucus Urethral culture: swab from 2-3 cm within the urethra Rectal culture: swab from 1 inch within the anal canal Oral culture: swab of the pharynx and tonsillar crypts
Heart scan; cardiac nuclear scanning; multiple gated acquisition (MUGA) scan; myocardial scan; nitroglycerin scan; pyrophosphate (PYP) heart scan; thallium	To assess for occurrence, extent, and prognosis of myocardial infarction; to monitor effectiveness of angioplasty coronary artery grafts; to assess myocardial wall abnormalities; to	Injection of radiopharmaceu-tical followed by nuclear imaging

Name/ Synonyms	Indication(s)	Description/ Specimen
scan; thallium stress testing	assess effect of nitroglycerin on ventricular function	
Hematocrit (Hct); crit; packed cell volume (PCV)	To assess the extent of blood loss and of normal hydration levels	Blood sample
Hemoglobin electrophoresis (Hgb electro- phoresis)	To identify abnormal types or amounts of hemoglobin	Blood sample
Hepatitis antigens and antibodies; hepatitis A; hepatitis B; hepatitis C; Deltavirus	To assess for inflammation of the liver caused by virus, bacteria, or toxic substance	Blood sample
Herpes simplex antibody, herpes genitalis, herpes simplex virus (HSV), herpesvirus	To assess for the herpes simplex virus	Blood sample
High-density lipoprotein (HDL)	To assess for high-density lipoprotein in the blood	Blood sample
Human immuno-deficiency virus (HIV) testing; acquired immu-nodeficiency	To assess for human immunodeficiency virus	Blood sample

Name/ Synonyms	Indication(s)	Description/ Specimen
syndrome (AIDS) test; AIDS serology; ELISA for HIV and antibody; HIV antibody test; Western blot for HIV and antibody		
Human leukocyte antigen test (HLA test); HLA typing; tissue typing	To determine tissue compatibility (organ transplantation) and paternity testing	Blood sample
5-Hydroxyindoleacetic acid (5-HIAA)	To identify the presence of carcinoid tumors of the intestine	Urine sample
Immunoelectrophoresis; antibodies; gamma globulins; immunoglobulins (IgA, IgD, IgE, IgG, IgM)	To measure immunoglobulins in the blood	Blood sample
Immunoglobulin light chain; Bence Jones protein	To assess for multiple myeloma and amyloidosis	Urine sample
Insulin; insulin assay; serum insulin	To assess the level of insulin in the serum	Blood sample

Name/ Synonyms	Indication(s)	Description/ Specimen
Iron (Fe)	To assess for anemia	Blood sample
Kidneys, ureters, and bladder radiography (KUB); flat plate x-ray of the abdomen; scout film	To provide an overall view of the lower abdomen; to assess for renal enlargement or displacement, congenital anomalies, renal or ureteral calculi, or ascites and gas in the intestine	X-ray film
Lactic acid; blood lactate	To assess for liver disease	Blood sample
Lactic dehydrogenase and isoenzymes; lactate dehydrogenase (LDH, LD)	To assess for myocardial infarction, biliary obstruction, bone metastases, cancer of prostate, hepatitis, liver damage, macrocytic anemia, pneumonia, muscular dystrophy, shock, or trauma	Blood sample
Lactose tolerance test	To assess for lactose intolerance	Blood sample
Laparoscopy; gynecologic	To assess pelvic pain for carcinoma, ectopic pregnancy, endometriosis,	Insertion of a laparoscope

Name/ Synonyms	Indication(s)	Description/ Specimen
laparoscopy; pelvic endoscopy; pelviscopy; peritoneoscopy	pelvic inflammatory disease (PID), and pelvic masses; to view fallopian tubes; to perform lysis of adhesions, ovarian biopsy and tubal ligation	through a small subumbilical incision for visualization and performance of procedures
Lipase	To assess abdominal pain	Blood sample
Lipid profile	To evaluate coronary heart disease risk	Usually includes high-density lipoprotein cholesterol, low-density lipoprotein cholesterol, triglycerides, and total cholesterol tests
Liver and pancreatobiliary system ultrasonography; gallbladder and biliary system sonogram; liver sonogram; pancreas sonogram	To assess for jaundice, hepatomegaly, abdominal trauma, cholecystectomy, metastatic tumors of the liver, or pancreatic carcinoma; to guide needle biopsy	Ultrasound waves are sent into the body with a small transducer pressed against the skin
Liver biopsy; percutaneous	To assess for disease of the liver, elevated liver	

Name/Synonyms	Indication(s)	Description/Specimen
liver biopsy; percutaneous needle biopsy of the liver	enzymes, jaundice, hepatomegaly, or possible rejection of a transplanted liver	An aspirated sample of liver tissue
Low-density lipoprotein (LDL)	To assess for low-density lipoprotein in the blood	Blood sample
Lung biopsy	To determine malignancy of a lung mass	An aspirated sample of lung mass tissue
Lung scan; lung perfusion scan; lung ventilation scan; ventilation/perfusion scanning	To detect pulmonary emboli and assess arterial perfusion of the lungs	Perfusion: A radiopharmaceutical is injected; scintillation camera is positioned over the chest Ventilation: Radioactive gas is inhaled through a face mask and the chest is scanned
Lupus erythematosus test (LE test); LE cell prep	To assess for lupus erythematosus	Blood sample
Luteinizing hormone (LH)	To determine whether ovulation occurred; to assess amenorrhea and infertility	Blood sample

Name/ Synonyms	Indication(s)	Description/ Specimen
Lyme disease antibody test	To evaluate for Lyme disease	Blood sample
Lymphangio-graphy; lymphography	To detect and stage lymphomas and assist in diagnosis	Injection of contrast medium, fluoroscopic visualization, and radiographic films
Magnesium	To assess magnesium level in the blood	Blood sample
Magnetic resonance imaging (MRI)	To evaluate cerebral infarct, abnormalities of the brain and spine, knee injuries, arteriovenous malformation, congenital heart disease, dementia, glomerulonephritis, hydronephrosis, multiple sclerosis, osteomyelitis, seizures, or spinal cord injuries	Imaging while in the MRI cylinder
Mammography	Routine screening for tumors	X-ray film of the breast
Mediastinoscopy	To assess for lymphoma, sarcoidosis, staging of lung cancer	Direct visualization of the contents of the mediastinum via a mediastinoscope inserted at the suprasternal notch.

Name/ Synonyms	Indication(s)	Description/ Specimen
Mononucleosis test; Epstein-Barr virus (EBV) antibody test; heterophil antibody titer (HAT); infectious mononucleosis testing; Monospot test	To assess for infectious mononucleosis	Blood sample
Myelography	To assess the subarachnoid space of the spinal column for tumors, bone structure changes, or herniations of intervertebral disks	Injection of contrast dye; visualization via fluoroscopy
Osmolality; serum/urine osmolality	To assess fluid and electrolyte imbalance, fluid requirements, urine concentration, and antidiuretic hormone (ADH) secretion, and for toxicology workups	Blood or urine sample
Oximetry; ear oximetry; pulse oximetry; oxygen saturation (SaO$_2$)	To monitor the oxygen saturation of arterial blood	A sensor emits beams of light through the skin tissue; rate and amount of

Name/ Synonyms	Indication(s)	Description/ Specimen
		absorption is converted to percentage of oxygen saturation present in the blood and is shown on monitor
Papanicolaou smear (Pap smear); exfoliative cytologic study; Pap test	To detect cervical cancer	Vaginal speculum is used to collect secretions from the cervix and endocervical canal
Paracentesis; abdominal paracentesis; abdominal tap; peritoneal fluid analysis; peritoneal tap	To determine cause of ascites or to remove ascites; to check for abdominal bleeding	Sample of fluid obtained through incision or needle
Parathyroid hormone (PTH); parathormone	To assist in differential diagnosis of parathyroid disorder	Blood sample
Partial thromboplastin time (PTT); activated partial thromboplastin time (APTT)	To detect bleeding disorders	Blood sample
Phosphorus (P); phosphate (PO_4)	To assess phosphorus level	Blood sample

Name/ Synonyms	Indication(s)	Description/ Specimen
Platelet count; thrombocyte count	To assess for thrombocytopenia, thrombocytosis, and platelet production	Blood sample
Pleural biopsy	To determine the nature of pleural tissue	Pleural tissue aspirated through a needle
Positron emission tomography (PET); single photon emission computed tomography (SPECT)	To study blood flow and metabolic changes in organs or regions of body tissues	A radionuclide is administered via IV or inhalation with the patient within the PET scanner
Potassium, blood/urine	To assess potassium level in the blood	Blood sample
Pregnancy test; human chorionic gonadotropin (hCG)	To determine pregnancy	Blood sample
Proctosigmoido-scopy; anoscopy; proctoscopy; sigmoidoscopy	To assess lower abdominal pain, change in bowel habits, and passage of blood, mucus or pus in the stool	The sigmoido-scope is inserted into the anus and advanced into the distal sigmoid colon; the sigmoid colon, rectum and anus are visualized

Name/ Synonyms	Indication(s)	Description/ Specimen
Progesterone	To assess the level of progesterone in the blood	Blood sample
Prostate-specific antigen (PSA)	To assess for prostate cancer, monitor its progression, or monitor response to prostate cancer treatment	Blood sample
Protein C (PC)	To evaluate severe thrombosis	Blood sample
Protein electrophoresis; serum protein electrophoresis (SPEP)	To evaluate albumin and each of the globulins	Blood sample
Protein; total protein (TP); albumin; alpha globulins; beta globulins; gamma globulins	To assess level of protein in the blood	Blood sample
Prothrombin time (PT); PT ratio/ INR; pro time	To evaluate the coagulation process	Blood sample
Pulmonary function tests (PFTs); spirometry	To measure pulmonary volume and capacity	Mouth-breathing into a spirometer as directed for readings of lung capacity and volume

Name/ Synonyms	Indication(s)	Description/ Specimen
Pyruvate kinase (PK)	To assess the level of pyruvate kinase in the blood; to assess for hemolytic anemia	Blood sample
Red blood cell count (RBC count); erythrocyte count	To measure the number of red blood cells per cubic millimeter of blood	Blood sample
Red blood cell indices (RBC indices); blood indices; mean corpuscular hemoglobin (MCH), mean corpuscular hemoglobin concentration (MCHC); mean corpuscular volume (MCV)	To determine normal size and amount of red blood cells	Blood sample
Renal biopsy; kidney biopsy	To assist in diagnosis of renal parenchymal disease	Renal tissue sample obtained through surgical incision or needle aspiration
Renal scan; kidney scan	To detect renal infarct, renal arterial atherosclerosis, renal trauma, renal tumor or cyst, or	Radiopharmaceutical administered by injection; scintillation camera is positioned over

Name/ Synonyms	Indication(s)	Description/ Specimen
	primary renal disease	the right upper quadrant
Reticulocyte count (retic count)	To assist in differential diagnosis of anemia	Blood sample
Retrograde pyelography; pyelography	To assess for bladder tumor, hydronephrosis, polycystic kidney disease, ureteral calculi, or renal cysts	Radiopaque iodine-based contrast medium is injected through a catheter into each kidney; radiographic films are taken of the ureters
Rheumatoid factor (RF); rheumatoid arthritis (RA) factor	To assess for rheumatoid arthritis	Blood test
Scrotal ultrasound; ultrasound of testes	To assess for scrotal masses and infection; to evaluate scrotal pain; to locate undescended testicles	A transducer is placed on the skin and moved as needed to provide visualization of the scrotal contents
Semen analysis; seminal cytology; sperm count	Used in fertility workup	Semen specimen

Name/ Synonyms	Indication(s)	Description/ Specimen
Skeletal x-ray; bone x-ray; sella turcica x-ray; skeletal radiography; skull x-ray; spinal x-ray; vertebral x-ray	To assess for bone deformities, fractures, dislocations, tumors, or metabolic abnormalities	Radiographic films of specific area
Sodium	To assess sodium level in the blood	Blood or urine sample
Sputum culture and sensitivity (sputum C&S)	To diagnose bacterial, fungal, or nonbacterial lower respiratory tract pneumonia	Sputum sample
Stool culture; stool for ova and parasites	To identify pathogens in the GI tract	Stool sample
Stool for occult blood; Hematest; Hemoccult (guaiac)	To identify blood in the GI tract	Stool sample
Syphilis serology; fluorescent treponemal antibody absorption (FTA-ABS); microhe-magglutination-Treponema pallidum (MHA-TP); rapid	To assess for Treponema pallidum	Blood sample

Name/ Synonyms	Indication(s)	Description/ Specimen
plasma reagin (RPR); Venereal Disease Research Laboratory (VDRL)		
T- and B-cell lymphocyte counts; acquired immunodeficiency syndrome (AIDS) T-lymphocyte cell markers; CD4 marker; T- and B-cell lymphocyte surface markers	To assess for Graves disease, viral infection, human immunodeficiency virus (HIV) infection, risk of AIDS, measles, or Hodgkin disease	Blood sample
Testosterone	To assess testosterone level in blood	Blood sample
Thoracentesis; pleural fluid analysis; pleural tap	To determine the cause of fluid production in the lungs	Aspiration of pleural fluid via a needle
Throat culture and sensitivity	To assess for pathogens	Swab of the tonsillar area and posterior pharynx
Thyroid scan	To assess size, shape, position, and function of the thyroid gland	IV administration of radioactive trace; scanning with scintillation camera

Name/ Synonyms	Indication(s)	Description/ Specimen
Thyroid-stimulating hormone (TSH); thyrotropin	To assess thyroid hormone levels	Blood sample
Thyroxine (T_4); total T_4	To assess thyroid hormone levels	Blood sample
Thyroxine free; free t_4 (ft_4)	To assess thyroid hormone levels	Blood sample
Total carbon dioxide content; carbon dioxide content (CO_2 content)	To assess carbon dioxide level in the blood	Blood sample
Total iron-binding capacity (TIBC)	To assess the maximum amount of iron that can be bound to transferrin	Blood sample
Toxicology screen; drug screen	To determine cause of drug toxicity, monitor compliance, and detect presence of drugs for employment or legal purposes	Blood or urine specimen
Transesophageal echocardiography (TEE)	To evaluate thoracic, aortic, and cardiac disorders	Gastroscope introduced into the mouth and advanced to the level of the right atrium of the heart; sound waves from the

Name/ Synonyms	Indication(s)	Description/ Specimen
		transducer on the gastroscope are transformed into a visual display
Transferrin; iron-binding protein; siderophilin	To assess the level of transferrin	Blood sample
Triglycerides	To assess triglyceride level	Blood sample
Triiodothyronine (T_3); total T_3	To assess thyroid hormone levels	Blood sample
Triiodothyronine uptake test (T_3 uptake); T_3 resin uptake	To assess thyroid hormone levels	Blood sample
Tuberculin (TB) skin test; Mantoux test; purified protein derivative (PPD) skin test; tine test	To screen for previous infection by tubercle bacillus	Intradermal injection of purified protein derivatives (PPDs)
Upper gastrointestinal and small bowel series; gastric radiography; small bowel study; stomach x-ray; upper GI series	To assess dysphagia, regurgitation, burning epigastric pain, hematemesis, melena, or weight loss	Barium is ingested while fluoroscopic films are taken of the esophagus, stomach, and small intestine

Name/ Synonyms	Indication(s)	Description/ Specimen
Urea nitrogen, blood urea nitrogen (BUN); urinary urea nitrogen	To assess the level of urea nitrogen	Blood or urine sample
Uric acid	To assess for uric acid	Blood or urine sample
Urinalysis (UA); routine urinalysis	Routine screening in physical examination, preoperative testing, hospital admission for diagnosis of infection of the kidneys and urinary tract, and diseases unrelated to the urinary system	Urine sample
Urine culture and sensitivity (urine for C&S)	To identify the specific bacterial organism present in the urine	Urine sample
Uroflowmetry; urine flow studies; urodynamic studies	To detect dysfunctional voiding patterns	Urination into a flowmeter to measure duration, amount, and rate
Urography; infusion	To demonstrate normal anatomy and wide range of	IV administration of contrast material, which is excreted by the kidneys;

Name/ Synonyms	Indication(s)	Description/ Specimen
pyelogram; intravenous pyelogram (IVP)	abnormalities involving the urinary tract	radiographs are exposed for evaluation of the morphology and function of the urinary tract
Vanillylmandelic acid and catecholamines (VMA); dopamine; epinephrine; norepinephrine; metanephrine; normetanephrine	To assess for neuroblastoma, stress, idiopathic orthostatic hypertension, and pheochromocytoma	Urine sample
Vitamin B_{12}; cyanocobalamin; extrinsic factor	To assess for macrocytic anemia	Blood sample
White blood cell (WBC) count and differential; basophil count; eosinophil count; leukocyte count; lymphocyte count; monocyte count; neutrophil count	To assess the total number of white blood cells and percentage of differentiation	Blood sample
Wound culture and sensitivity	To identify the specific bacterial organism present in the wound	Swab of the wound site

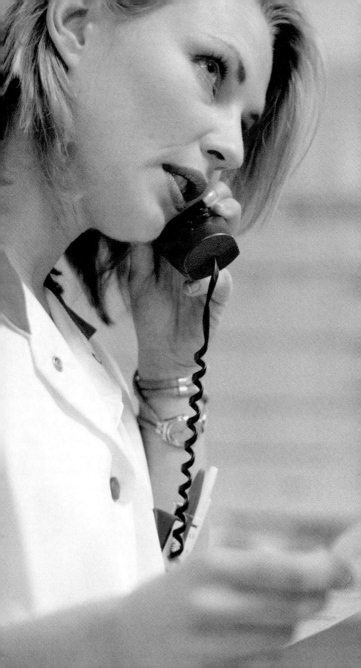

Medical Records

The information contained in the patient's medical record is used to assess previous treatment, to ensure continuity of care, and to avoid unnecessary tests or procedures. These documents also create a legal record that benefits the patient and his or her healthcare providers. A patient's medical record can be an invaluable tool for healthcare providers, but to live up to its full potential, the different parts of the medical record must be as complete and as accurate as possible.

General Guidelines

Although every hospital or office has specific policies regarding the placement of various portions of text on the page, the following guidelines concerning the format and style of the documents that comprise a patient's medical record should prove acceptable in most situations.

Page Numbering

Page numbers help keep reports in correct page order.

- Pages are numbered consecutively.
- Page numbers can appear in the top or bottom of the document and can be aligned at the left, center, or right margin.
- Generally, the first page of a document is not numbered.
- The number can be part of the document text, or it may appear in the document's header or footer.

Headings

Section headings are used to document the evaluation and management of a patient in a logical fashion. A typical medical report contains most or all of the following section headings, or a variation of them, which outline the patient's history, diagnosis, and plan of care:

- **Chief Complaint (CC):** States the specific reason the patient sought medical care.

- **History of Present Illness (HPI):** Documents the complete story of why the patient is seeking medical attention. It is usually arranged in chronological order beginning with the earliest relevant facts and proceeding to the point where the patient was admitted or seen in an office visit.

- **Past Medical History:** Includes information about the patient's previous illnesses, injuries, or chronic conditions.

- **Past Surgical History:** Contains information about past surgical procedures the patient has undergone.

- **Medications:** Lists the medications that the patient is currently taking and the dosages of each.

- **Allergies:** Lists the patient's allergies. Some physicians also dictate sensitivities to foods or other items here, such as rashes that may result from seafood or latex.

- **Family History:** Outlines information about hereditary or family illnesses, and provides evidence for considering that the patient may be suffering from those diseases, as well as infections or contagious illnesses to which the patient may be exposed.

- **Social History:** Details a patient's marital status and work and living situation, and may also include social habits such as smoking, alcohol use, or illicit drug use.

- **Review of Systems (ROS):** Contains a brief overall review of the medical condition of the patient's body organs systems, which may or may not be relevant to the HPI. The systems review may be contained in one paragraph, or may be subdivided into separate categories (such as pulmonary, cardiovascular, gastrointestinal, genitourinary, musculoskeletal, lymphatic, skin, hematologic, neurologic, and/or psychiatric).

- **Physical Examination (PE):** Outlines the physician's thorough examination of the patient, including observations and findings. The physical exam section may be written in paragraph form, or may be laid out using subheadings. The subsections of the PE are addressed in a standard order from head to toe. They can appear in paragraph form after the main heading, or as subheadings flush left under the main heading. These subsections may include the following:

  - **Vital Signs (VS):** Indicates the patient's vital signs such as temperature, blood pressure, pulse, respirations, height, and weight. Extra items such as body mass index (BMI) or oxygen saturation might also be indicated here.

  - **General Appearance:** Indicates the general appearance of the patient, such as physical build, personal hygiene, and mood.

  - **HEENT:** Denotes the findings of the head, eyes, ears, nose, and throat.

  - **Neck:** Palpated for abnormal enlargement of lymph nodes or jugular veins, or abnormal carotid artery pulses.

  - **Lungs:** Indicates the amount and quality of air moving in and out of the lungs as evaluated by auscultation through a stethoscope.

- **Heart:** Reveals abnormal sounds associated with the beating heart such as murmurs or rubs that are heard through a stethoscope.

- **Abdomen:** Indicates abnormal bowel sounds or tenderness, guarding, or masses in the abdominal region, including the liver and spleen.

- **Extremities:** Specifies findings related to blood flow to the extremities, such as dorsalis pedis and posterior tibial pulses as well as capillary refill. This section also denotes findings related to developmental or traumatic deformities of the extremities.

- **Neurologic:** Details findings related to the nervous system, including motor strength and sensation of the extremities, mental status, and functioning of the cranial nerves and reflexes.

- **Laboratory Data:** Includes information about the results of laboratory and diagnostic tests.

- **Assessment and Plan:** Details the physician's findings and diagnoses based on the information already presented and outlines a treatment plan, including procedures and their rationale, and plans for following the course of the patient's illness. The assessment and plan may appear together as one heading, or be divided into two separate headings.

Signature

All medical reports contain at least one signature. The signature of the physician who will sign the report may be entered manually or electronically. Additional signature lines for dictating physicians may also be included. It is common practice to include the initials of the physician who dictated the report, along with the dictator's and transcriptionist's initials underneath the signature line, as well as the dates of the dictation and transcription of the report.

Types of Medical Reports

Patients are assessed continuously throughout their care by different medical providers. This assessment and reassessment process is documented in different types of reports, including clinic notes, history and physical reports, operative reports, consultation reports, discharge summaries, radiology reports, and pathology reports.

Clinic Note

A physician dictates a clinic note after every encounter with the patient. The note contains a reason for the visit, the supporting information about the presenting problem, the findings on physical examination, and a plan of treatment. The clinic note is usually short (only a few paragraphs), but some more extensive notes may carry over into subsequent pages. The note usually contains headings to separate the findings and help make them more readable.

Sample Clinic Note

Patient Name: Hasad Hussein
Medical Record Number: 90-45-622
Date of Service: 11/09/20xx

REASON FOR VISIT: Follow-up of obstructive sleep apnea.

HISTORY OF PRESENT ILLNESS: The patient has been on CPAP for approximately 1 year and no longer feels it is benefiting him. He still reports significant daytime sleepiness. He had septal surgery approximately last year with no relief. He is scheduled for a sleep study at our hospital next week. Previous sleep studies done at an outside hospital showed an apnea-hypopnea index of 33.6 per hour. Otherwise the patient is without complaints today.

PHYSICAL EXAMINATION:
GENERAL: This is a healthy-appearing male in no acute distress.
HEENT: There is no facial weakness. His voice is strong. There is no evidence of stridor. His ear canals are clear and tympanic membranes are intact. His nasal septum is midline. His turbinates are within normal limits bilaterally. There are no lesions or masses in the oral cavity or oropharynx. His tonsils are normal in size.
NECK: There is no palpable lymphadenopathy.
NEUROLOGIC: His cranial nerves are grossly intact.

ASSESSMENT: Obstructive sleep apnea.

PLAN: Based on the fact that the patient has a long history of sleep apnea, uvulopalatopharyngoplasty has been scheduled. We will defer the details of the surgery until the patient returns to clinic after his sleep study next week. He will follow up with us next month to discuss the details of the surgery and do final surgery scheduling.

Carol Anne Connors, MD[i]
CAC/xx
D: 11/09/20xx
T: 11/09/20xx

Some clinic notes follow a generalized formatting style called SOAP, which is an acronym for Subjective, Objective, Assessment, and Plan. A clinic note using the SOAP format, as shown below, is similar in appearance to that of other notes, except that the headings used in the note are simply Subjective, Objective, Assessment, and Plan. Each heading is described as follows:

- **Subjective:** Details the reason for the patient's visit and the immediate history behind the visit.

- **Objective:** Sets out the physical examination findings and results of laboratory or other diagnostic tests performed with regard to the patient's problem.

- **Assessment:** Contains the physician's discussion of the diagnosis based on the information presented.

- **Plan:** Indicates the treatment plan developed by the physician, given the patient's diagnostic assessment in the report, and plans for further followup, if applicable.

Sample SOAP Clinic Note

Patient Name: Andrew Jones
Medical Record Number: AJ12345
Date of Service: 03/03/20xx

S: This 36-year-old male returns for regular monthly refills on his medication for lumbar radiculitis. He had several lumbar surgeries related to a motor vehicle accident 3 years ago. He is stable on medication which includes methadone 30 mg b.i.d. and Lortab 7.5 mg t.i.d.

O: No acute distress. Blood pressure 117/73, heart rate 69, and he is afebrile with a temperature of 97.4. Lungs are clear. Heart is regular rate and rhythm. He is using a cane. Examination of the back shows lumbar concerns are stable.

A: Chronic pain. Lumbar radiculitis.

P: Medication agreement is in his chart. Refill on his medications as above. Return to clinic in 2 months and as needed.

Thomas L. Mansford, MD
TLM/xx
D: 03/03/20xx
T: 03/03/20xx

History and Physical Report

A history and physical examination (also called an H&P) is dictated by an attending physician when a patient is admitted to the hospital. It is the starting point of the patient's inpatient care and contains a summary of the patient's information known at the time of admission, including the problem or reason for admission, history of the present illness, a review of systems, and the patient's prior history. The physical examination portion includes a thorough examination, both subjective and objective, by the provider to assess the patient's condition in order to formulate an assessment and plan for treatment during the hospital stay.

Sample History and Physical

Patient Name: Jose Manuel Aguillar
Medical Record Number: 988-23100
Date of Admission: 07/15/20xx
Attending Physician: Eduardo G. Marcos, MD

CHIEF COMPLAINT: Fistula.

HISTORY OF PRESENT ILLNESS: The patient is a 48-year-old male with past medical history significant for gluten intolerance and rectal prolapse who subsequently underwent LAR and sphincteroplasty. His postoperative course has been complicated by the development of a fistula, and he is to undergo a fistulotomy in the morning with Dr. Beard. He denies any complaints with bowel movements. No blood per rectum. He has had two formed soft bowel movements every day; however, he did note some minimal pain at the fistula site.

PHYSICAL EXAMINATION ON ADMISSION:
VITAL SIGNS: Blood pressure 110/80, pulse 79, respirations 16, and temperature 98.6.
GENERAL: He is in no acute distress, alert and oriented ×3.
HEENT: Normocephalic, atraumatic. Extraocular muscles intact.
LUNGS: Clear to auscultation.
HEART: Normal S1, S2. No murmurs, rubs, or gallops.
ABDOMEN: Soft, nondistended and nontender. Normoactive bowel sounds.
EXTREMITIES: No clubbing, cyanosis, or edema.

LABORATORY DATA: White count 5.9, hematocrit 44.3, platelets 324, sodium 139, potassium 3.9, chloride 104, bicarb 28, BUN 14, creatinine 1.5, and glucose 101. Alkaline phosphatase 69, AST 19, ALT 23 and total bilirubin 1.

ASSESSMENT: The patient is a 48-year-old male with past medical history significant for rectal prolapse status post LAR and sphincteroplasty, now presenting with a fistula and is to undergo fistulotomy in the morning.

PLAN: Clear liquid diet today. The patient is n.p.o. after midnight. Check his preoperative labs, chest x-ray, and EKG.

Surgery consents are in the chart. Plans are for operative intervention in the morning.

_____

Eduardo G. Marcos, MD
EGM/xx
D: 03/03/20xx
T: 03/03/20xx

Operative Report

The operative report is dictated by the operating physician or assistant immediately after completion of a surgical procedure. It contains a detailed narrative of the procedure, including the preoperative and postoperative diagnoses, the type of procedure performed, the names of the surgeon(s) and attending nursing staff, the type of anesthesia and the name of the anesthesiologist, and other introductory details such as estimated blood loss, complications, materials left in the patient (such as pins, rods, or sutures), and intraoperative findings. A detailed description of the operative procedure itself follows and concludes with a disposition of the case or the location to which the patient was transferred after leaving the operating room.

Sample Operative Report

Patient Name: Sandra Mae Wilkinson
Medical Record Number: 472209
Date of Admission: 04/15/20xx
Attending Physician: Daniel Wang, MD

DATE OF PROCEDURE: April 20, 20xx.

PREOPERATIVE DIAGNOSIS: Respiratory insufficiency with retained secretions.

POSTOPERATIVE DIAGNOSIS: Respiratory insufficiency with retained secretions.

SURGEON: Daniel Wang, MD

ASSISTANT: Eugene Waller, MD

PROCEDURE PERFORMED: Mini-tracheostomy.

ESTIMATED BLOOD LOSS: Minimal.

ANESTHESIA: Monitored anesthesia care, local.

INDICATIONS FOR PROCEDURE: The patient is a 62-year-old female well known from the cardiothoracic surgery service with a history of pneumonia that was complicated with right upper lobe resection that was drained and treated in the past. The patient had a long and very complicated course with worsening of her respiratory status and respiratory failure. The patient had a large amount of secretions and required frequent suctioning, and it was decided to perform a mini-tracheostomy to facilitate the suctioning of the airway while allowing normal respirations through her own airway. The risks and benefits of the procedure were discussed with the patient and the daughter who agreed to the procedure and signed the consent.

DESCRIPTION OF PROCEDURE: The patient was taken to the operating room and placed in the supine position. After a minimal sedation was achieved, the area of the neck and upper chest was prepped and draped in sterile fashion. The area of the skin over the second and third tracheal cartilage was anesthetized with 2 mL of 1% lidocaine.

A 4-mm incision was made in the skin with a #11 blade. Over this incision, the trachea was accessed using a large-bore needle. A guide wire was introduced through the large-bore needle and the needle removed. Then a small dilator was introduced through the guide wire to enlarge the size of the stoma. The 4-mm mini-tracheostomy tube was inserted in the trachea. The guide wire and dilator were removed. The mini-tracheostomy tube was secured in place.

Sedation was reversed and the patient was awake, smiling, and following commands. The mini-tracheostomy was used for suctioning successfully. The patient was taken to the recovery room in stable condition.

_____

Daniel Wang, MD
DW/xx
D: 04/20/20xx
T: 04/20/20xx

Consultation Report

A consultation contains an expert second opinion about a patient's condition requested by the attending physician to aid in the diagnosis and treatment of the patient. The report is dictated by this second physician, called the consulting physician, and it generally includes the date and reason for the consultation, the objective evaluation of the patient, and the consultant's recommendations for treatment. The consultation may be dictated in a letter format to the attending physician or it can be dictated as a medical report and look similar in appearance and formatting as other reports. Both styles can contain subheadings such as History of Present Illness, Past History, Physical Examination, Impression, and Recommendations for Treatment.

Sample Consultation (Letter Format)

September 25, 20xx
Erika Lee Marcone, MD
4600 Van Buren Street
Nashville, TN 37213

Re: Patient: Christina Dorman
       MR Number: 987720-55

Dear Dr. Marcone:

Thank you for asking me to see your patient, Christina Dorman, for a second opinion regarding her vesicoureteral reflux. She is a 5-month-old white female, an ex-24-weeker who weighed 550 grams at birth, who has had multiple ultrasounds. Her first ultrasound demonstrated a fungus ball in the right renal pelvis. This resolved a month later and after aggressive diuretic therapy in the MICU, she developed nephrocalcinosis. Followup ultrasound demonstrated resolution of the calcinosis by demonstrating moderate left hydronephrosis. A VCUG was done to investigate this and demonstrated with a grade 3 reflux on the right and grade 4 reflux on the left. She has since been on amoxicillin prophylaxis and she has had had no infections.

Her past medical history is significant for prematurity, respiratory distress syndrome requiring prolonged intubation, GERD, stridor, recurrent pneumonias, retinopathy of prematurity, nephrocalcinosis, chronic lung disease, and cor pulmonale. She previously underwent a Nissen fundoplication, surgical G tube, bronchoscopy, and central line placement and exchange.

She takes amoxicillin 90 mg by mouth daily, Zantac, Diuril, and salt replacement. She has no known drug allergies.

On physical exam, her temperature is 97.8, heart rate 123, blood pressure 74/50, saturating 94% on room air. She is in no distress.

Her abdomen is soft, nontender, and nondistended. There are no palpable masses and her kidneys are not palpable bilaterally. Her G tube is in place in her left epigastric area. She has no CVA tenderness bilaterally to exam. She has normal external genitalia on the genital exam. No sacral dimple. She has wet diapers and no clubbing, cyanosis, or edema.

Her laboratory data shows a negative urine culture. Creatinine was 0.2 and BUN 16. Last white count was done on 06/20/05 and this was 22,000.

Assessment: This is a 5-month-old ex-24-weeker with bilateral vesicoureteral reflux.

Recommendations:

1. Continue amoxicillin prophylaxis. May change to Bactrim prophylaxis at this point as she is older than 6 weeks.

2. Follow up in 3 months with pediatric urology with Dr. Salim Lakshman. Call 615-955-6100 for an appointment and when she presents to this visit, she will be 8 months old and she should have a new ultrasound at that time.

3. When she is 12 months of age, she should follow up again and at that point receive an ultrasound, a voiding cystourethrogram, and a DMSA scan at that visit.

Thank you for asking me to participate in the care of your patient. If you have any questions or concerns, please do not hesitate to contact me.

Sincerely,
Danil Viktor, MD

DV/xx

Progress Note

A progress note is dictated during the patient's hospital stay and is created as often as the patient's condition warrants. The note relates to the patient's condition and progress, complications, response to treatment, and plan for immediate future treatment.

Sample Progress Note

Name of Patient: Santiago Panigua
Medical Record No.: 16174332
Date of Service: 07/31/20xx
Date of Admission: 07/22/20xx
Provider: Julia Michaud, MD

INTERVAL HOSPITAL COURSE: The patient received his methotrexate and rituximab without major complications. He is ambulating and he is eating. He is afebrile. His blood sugars continue to be high so he is on sliding scale with insulin coverage. We will continue with supportive care and close followup as well as his leucovorin.

_____

Dictated by: Julia Michaud, MD/394
D: 07/31/20xx
T: 08/01/20xx

Discharge Summary

A discharge summary is dictated by the attending physician for a patient who is discharged from the hospital. It summarizes the patient's course of treatment in the hospital, including tests and other workups performed, and pertinent physical findings throughout the course of the hospital stay. The report may also include discharge medications, discharge instructions, and follow-up information for the patient.

Sample Discharge Summary

Name of Patient: Jane Smith
Medical Record No.: 68821
Date of Admission: 08/02/20xx
Date of Discharge: 08/05/20xx
Attending Physician: Joseph D. McGraw, MD

DIAGNOSES

1. Lumbar spinal stenosis.

2. Hyperlordosis of the lumbar spine.

3. Postoperative anemia.

4. History of asthma.

PROCEDURES PERFORMED

1. Foraminotomy and laminectomy from L2-S1.

2. Posterior spinal fusion with instrumentation from T12-S1.

3. Iliac crest bone grafting of the right hip.

4. Packed red blood cell transfusion for postoperative anemia.

BRIEF HISTORY: The patient is a 50-year-old female who presented to her primary physician complaining of lower back pain, lower back deformity, and bilateral lower extremity pain.

Physical exam and radiographic workup was consistent with a diagnosis of hyperlordosis of the lumbar spine with associated spinal stenosis. Despite medical management, the patient continued to have pain and symptoms consistent with her diagnosis of spinal stenosis. She elected to undergo surgical treatment. Informed consent was obtained after the risks, benefits and potential complications were explained at length with the patient. She agreed and wished to proceed.

HOSPITAL COURSE: The patient was taken to the operating room where the above procedure was performed. Postoperatively the patient was admitted to the intensive care unit overnight and subsequently transferred to the floor. Her diet was gradually advanced with the return of bowel function. She began tolerating clear liquids and her Foley catheter and PCA pump were removed. Her drains from her surgical sites were removed when output was deemed minimal. On the second postoperative day, she was noted to have postoperative anemia. Therefore, she received a transfusion of packed red blood cells and ultimately thereafter, her hematocrit remained stable.

At the time of discharge, she was ambulating, weightbearing as tolerated, voiding with the use of a Foley catheter, told a regular diet, and pain was adequately controlled with oral pain medications. In addition, she was afebrile with stable vital signs and her white count and hematocrit. Her incision was clean and dry without evidence of infection and she was neurologically intact.

DISCHARGE MEDICATIONS

1. Oxycodone 5–10 mg every 4–6 hours as needed for pain.

2. Colace 100 mg b.i.d. while on oxycodone.

DISCHARGE INSTRUCTIONS

1. Diet: Regular diet.

2. Activity: Weightbearing as tolerated.

FOLLOW-UP INSTRUCTIONS: The patient should follow up with her primary physician in 2 weeks. The patient should notify her physician of any fevers greater than 101.5, any redness or discharge from the wound, any increased or uncontrolled pain, or any other questions or concerns.

_____

Joseph D. McGraw, MD
JDM/xx
D: (Current Date)
T: (Current Date)

Radiology Report

The radiology report is dictated by a radiologist, who reviews and interprets images obtained from x-rays, CT scans, MRI scans, ultrasounds, and other radiologic modalities and issues a report of the findings to the requesting physician. The report typically includes the date of the evaluation, type of test, and a "read" of the image to pinpoint an injury or help detect abnormalities such as masses or tumors, along with the radiologist's impression or diagnosis of the findings.

Sample Radiology Report

Patient Name: Lorena Jones
Medical Record Number: HW-4922L
Date of Admission: 06/27/xx
Attending Physician: Hyatt Mullen, MD

DATE OF EVALUATION: June 20, 20xx

ORDERING PHYSICIAN: Hyatt Mullen, MD

TYPE OF TEST: X-ray evaluation.

INDICATION: Cardiac palpitations.

FINDINGS: The lungs show essentially mild increase in interstitial markings. The cardiac silhouette is enlarged. The costophrenic angles are clear. Hilar regions are within upper limits of normal in size.

IMPRESSION: Mildly increased interstitial markings in the lung fields which represent mild component of venous congestion. Follow-up examination is recommended. The cardiac silhouette is within upper limits of normal in size.

Richard Moore, MD
Attending Radiologist
RM/gnw
T: 06/28/xx
D: 06/28/xx

Pathology Report

The pathology report is dictated by a pathologist who describes findings relating to disease and/or pathology of tissue sample submitted as a result of a surgery, special procedure, or biopsy. The pathologist studies the cells of the tissue and renders a diagnosis based on the gross and microscopic findings that helps to provide a foundation for the patient's treatment. The findings are rendered in the form of a pathology report addressed to the requesting physician.

Sample Pathology Report

Date: 12/06/xx
Pathology No.: M02-3551
Reg. No.: 000038
Patient Name: Sally M. Goodwin
Medical Record No. 70783220

HISTORY: Multiple transurethral resections of bladder for grade II transitional cell carcinoma; multiple tumors.

GROSS DESCRIPTION: The specimen is received in two parts. They are labeled #1, "biopsy bladder tumor," and #2, "scalene node, left." Part #1 consists of multiple fragments of gray-brown tissue which appear slightly hemorrhagic. Part #2 consists of multiple fragments of fatty yellow tissue which range in size from 0.2 to 1 cm in diameter.

MICROSCOPIC DESCRIPTION: Section of bladder contains areas of transitional cell carcinoma. No area of invasion can be identified. A marked acute and chronic inflammatory reaction with eosinophils is noted together with some necrosis. Section of lymph node contains normal node with reactive germinal centers.

DIAGNOSES

1. Papillary transitional cell carcinoma, grade 2, bladder biopsy.

2. Acute and chronic inflammation, most consistent with recent biopsy procedure.

3. Scalene lymph node, left, no pathologic diagnosis.

COMMENT: This transitional cell carcinoma is well differenti-
ated. Tissue has been sent for immunohistochemical studies.
These results will be issued as an addendum.

_____

Lai Chei Nguyen, MD
Pathologist

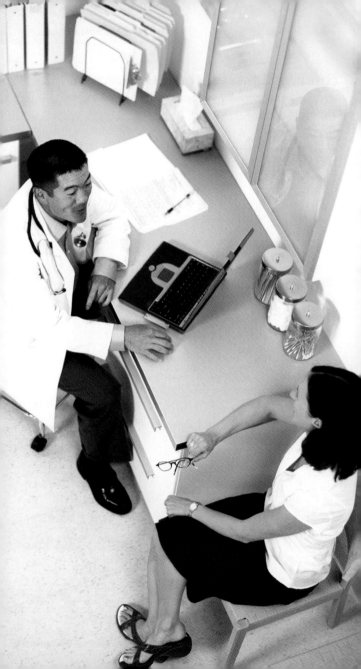

Internet Resources

General

Aurora Healthcare http://www.aurorahealthcare.org/yourhealth/
healthgate/getcontent.asp?URLhealthgate=45979.html

Centers for Medicare & Medicaid Services (CMS) (HHS
agency responsible for administering Medicare, Medicaid, and
the Health Insurance Portability and Accountability Act [HIPPA])
http://www.cms.hhs.gov

eMedicine.com http://www.emedicine.com

Institute for Safe Medication Practices http://www.ismp.org/

**Joint Commission on Accreditation of Healthcare
Organizations** http://www.jcaho.org/

Lab Tests Online (public resource on clinical laboratory
testing) http://www.labtestsonline.org/

Medline Plus http://medlineplus.gov/

Medline Plus (drugs, supplements, and herbals information)
http://www.nlm.nih.gov/medlineplus/druginformation.html

OR-Live http://www.or-live.com/archives.cfm

Radiology Info (resource explaining radiologic procedures and therapies) http://www.radiologyinfo.org/

Rx List (drug information) http://www.rxlist.com

U.S. Department of Health and Human Services (HHS)
http://www.hhs.gov/

U.S. Food and Drug Administration http://www.fda.org

United States Pharmacopeia (sets standards to ensure the quality of medicines) http://www.usp.org

Alternative and Complementary Medicine

Alternative Health News Online http://www.altmedicine.com

The Alternative Medicine Homepage
http://www.pitt.edu/~cbw/altm.html

Alternative Medicine Magazine
http://www.naturalsolutionmag.com

American Association for Health Freedom
http://www.apma.net

American Botanical Council http://www.herbalgram.org

American College of Occupational and Environmental Medicine http://www.acoem.org

American Herbalists Guild
http://www.americanherbalistsguild.com

American Herbal Pharmacopoeia http://www.herbal-ahp.org

American Herbal Products Association http://www.ahpa.org

The American Holistic Medical Association
http://www.holisticmedicine.org

American Pain Foundation http://www.painfoundation.org

The American Society of Pharmacognosy
http://www.phcog.org

Ayurvedic Foundations http://www.ayur.com

Estronaut http://www.estronaut.com

Health Action Network Society http://www.hans.org

HealthWorld Online http://www.healthy.net

The Herb Society of America http://www.herbsociety.org

HerbMed http://www.herbmed.org

Homeopathy Home http://www.homeopathyhome.com

The Institute for Traditional Medicine http://www.itmonline.org

**The International Association for the Study of Traditional
Asian Medicine** http://www.iastam.org/home.htm

The International Register of Consultant Herbalists and Homeopaths http://www.irch.org

KidsHealth http://www.kidshealth.org

Mayo Clinic http://www.mayoclinic.com

National Center for Complementary and Alternative Medicine (National Institutes of Health) http://nccam.nih.gov

Naturopathic Medicine Network http://www.pandamedicine.com

Oncolink http://oncolink.upenn.edu

Reuters Health News http://www.reutershealth.com

Blood and Lymph

AIDS information http://www.aidsinfonyc.org

Aplastic anemia and MDS (myelodysplastic syndromes) http://www.aamds.org/aplastic/

Blood information http://www.bloodbook.com/index.html

Blood transfusion and surgery http://www.yoursurgery.com/proceduredetails.cfm?br=7&proc=7

The Body.com (AIDS and HIV information) http://www.thebody.com/index.html

Lab Tests Online http://www.labtestsonline.org/

Leukemia and Lymphoma Society
http://www.leukemia-lymphoma.org/hm_lls

Lymphoma Research Foundation
http://www.lymphoma.org/

National Heart, Lung and Blood Institute
http://www.NHLBI.nih.gov/

National Hemophilia Foundation (all bleeding disorders)
http://www.hemophilia.org/home.htm

Cardiology

American Heart Association http://www.americanheart.org/

American College of Cardiology http://www.acc.org

Angioplasty.org http://www.angioplasty.org

Cardiothoracic Surgery Network http://www.ctsnet.org/

Cardiothoracic Surgery Network Video Gallery
http://www.ctsnet.org/section/videogallery/

ECG Library http://www.ecglibrary.com

The Franklin Institute Online (heart basics)
http://www.fi.edu/learn/heart/index.html

The Heart.org http://www.theheart.org

Heart Surgery Forum
http://www.hsforum.com

Karolinska Institute
http://www.mic.ki.se/diseases/C14.html

Medical University of South Carolina (cardiovascular
perfusion) http://www.musc.edu/perfusion/interven.htm

Medtronic
http://www.medtronic.com/physician/cardiology.html

National Heart, Lung and Blood Institute
http://www.NHLBI.nih.gov/

PBS NOVA Cut to the Heart
http://www.pbs.org/wgbh/nova/heart/

St. Jude Medical Heart Library
http://www.heartlibrary.com/

University of California, San Diego, Medical Center
http://www.health.ucsd.edu/labref

Dermatology

Site sponsored by the American Academy of Dermatology
http://www.skincarephysicians.com/

Indiana University, Department of Dermatology Homepage
http://www.iupui.edu/~derm/home.html

Johns Hopkins University, Dermatology Image Atlas
http://dermatlas.med.jhmi.edu/derm/

Lupus Foundation of America
http://www.lupus.org/newsite/index.html

National Institute of Arthritis and Musculoskeletal and Skin Diseases (health information related to musculoskeletal and integumentary systems)
http://www.niams.nih.gov/hi/index.htm

The National Organization for Albinism and Hypopigmentation (NOAH) http://www.albinism.org/

Skin Cancer Foundation http://www.skincancer.org/

University of Iowa, Department of Dermatology Homepage
http://tray.dermatology.uiowa.edu/home.html

University of Iowa, Dermatologic Image Database
http://tray.dermatology.uiowa.edu/DermImag.htm

University of Texas South Western Medical Center at Dallas, Department of Dermatology, glossary of common skin diseases and therapies
http://www.swmed.edu/home_pages/derma/glossary.htm

Endocrinology

American Diabetes Association http://www.diabetes.org

Little People of America, Inc. (dwarfism information and support site) http://www.lpaonline.org/

National Adrenal Diseases Foundation
http://www.medhelp.org/nadf/

Pituitary Network Association http://www.pituitary.com/

Gastroenterology

American College of Gastroenterology—Patient Information Link http://www.acg.gi.org

American Society of Colon and Rectal Surgeons—Patient Education Link http://www.fascrs.org

Colon Cancer Alliance http://www.ccalliance.org/

Crohn's and Colitis Foundation of America
http://www.ccfa.org/

H. pylori **and ulcer** http://www.cdc.gov/ulcer/

United Ostomy Associations of America, Inc.
http://www.uoa.org/

Neurology

Alzheimer Association http://www.alz.org/

American Epilepsy Society http://www.aesnet.org/

American Sleep Apnea Association http://sleepapnea.org/

American Stroke Association http://www.strokeassociation.org/
presenter.jhtml?identifier=1200037

Epilepsy Foundation http://www.efa.org/index.cfm

Huntington's Disease Society of America
http://www.hdsa.org/

Hydrocephalus http://www.patientcenters.com/hydrocephalus/
news/whatishydro.html

Hydrocephalus Association http://www.hydroassoc.org/

Myasthenia Gravis Foundation of America, Inc.
http://www.myasthenia.org/

National Multiple Sclerosis Society http://www.nmss.org/

National Stroke Association http://www.stroke.org/

Parkinson's Disease Foundation
http://www.pdf.org/index.cfm

Spina Bifida Association http://www.sbaa.org/

Spine-Health
http://www.spine-health.com/dir/dir01.html#surgery

Whole Brain Atlas from Harvard Medical School
http://www.med.harvard.edu/AANLIB/home.html

Ophthalmology and Optometry

American Academy of Ophthalmology http://www.aao.org

American Optometric Association—Link to Eye Conditions
http://www.aoanet.org/

American Society of Cataract and Refractive Surgery
http://www.ascrs.org/

Eye Care America http://www.eyecareamerica.org/

LASIK Institute http://www.lasikinstitute.org/

Medem Medical Library—Eye Health
http://www.medem.com/medlb/
sub_detaillb.cfm?parent_id=30&act=disp

National Eye Institute http://www.nei.nih.gov/

Orthopaedics

American Academy of Orthopaedic Surgeons
http://www.aaos.org/

The American Orthopaedic Society for Sports Medicine
http://www.sportsmed.org

Arthritis Foundation http://www.arthritis.org/

Medical News Today
http://www.medicalnewstoday.com/sections/bones/

Muscular Dystrophy Association http://www.mdausa.org/

National Institute of Arthritis and Musculoskeletal and Skin Diseases http://www.niams.nih.gov/hi/index.htm

National Institutes of Health (osteoporosis and related bone diseases) http://www.osteo.org

National Osteoporosis Foundation http://www.nof.org/

Orthopaedics.com http://www.orthopaedics.com/

Scoliosis Research Society http://www.srs.org/

Southern California Orthopaedic Institute
http://www.scoi.com/

University of Washington Orthopaedics and Sports Medicine http://www.orthop.washington.edu/

Wayne State School of Medicine http://www.med.wayne.edu/diagRadiology/RSNA2003/Overview.htm

Wheeless' Textbook of Orthopaedics presented by Duke Orthopaedics http://www.wheelessonline.com/

Otology and Related Sites

American Academy of Otolaryngology http://www.entnet.org/

American Speech-Language-Hearing Association
http://www.asha.org/

National Institute on Deafness and Other Communication Disorders http://www.nidcd.nih.gov/

Psychiatry

American Psychiatric Association http://www.psych.org

Autism Society of America http://www.autism-society.org/

National Association of Anorexia Nervosa and Associated Disorders http://www.anad.org/

National Attention Deficit Association http://www.add.org/

National Depressive and Manic Depressive Association
http://ndmda.org/

National Institute of Mental Health http://www.nimh.nih.gov

Schizophrenia http://www.schizophrenia.com/

Reproductive Health

American College of Obstetrics and Gynecology—Patient Education http://www.acog.org/

American Society of Plastic & Reconstructive Surgeons (breast augmentation) http://www.plasticsurgery.org

American Society of Reproductive Medicine
http://www.asrm.com

American Urological Association—Patient info
http://www.auanet.org/

Center for Disease Control and Prevention (sexually transmitted diseases) http://www.cdc.gov/

OncoLink (prostate or testicular cancer)
http://www.oncolink.com/

Testicular Cancer Resource Center
http://tcrc.acor.org/index.html

Breast Cancer

OncoLink http://www.oncolink.com/

Susan G. Komen Breast Cancer Foundation
http://www.komen.org/

Respiratory Care

American Academy of Allergy, Asthma and Immunology
http://www.aaaai.org/

American Association for Respiratory Care (professional site for respiratory care including career description, patient education link) http://www.aarc.org/

American Lung Association http://www.lungusa.org/

American Sleep Apnea Association http://sleepapnea.org/

The Auscultation Assistant
http://www.wilkes.med.ucla.edu/lungintro.htm

It's Time to Focus on Lung Cancer site
http://www.lungcancer.org/

The National Emphysema Foundation
http://www.emphysemafoundation.org/

National Heart, Lung and Blood Institute
http://www.NHLBI.nih.gov/

The R.A.L.E. Repository http://www.rale.ca/

Urinology

American Urological Association—Patient info
http://www.auanet.org/

American Urologic Association Foundation
http://www.auafoundation.org/

Lab Tests Online (public resource on clinical laboratory testing) http://www.labtestsonline.org/

National Kidney Foundation http://www.kidney.org/

United Ostomy Association (urostomy [urinary diversion] information) http://www.uoa.org

UrologyHealth.org http://www.urologyhealth.org

Anatomy Atlas

Anterior and posterior views of the skull

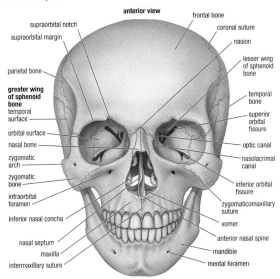

anterior view

- supraorbital notch
- supraorbital margin
- parietal bone
- **greater wing of sphenoid bone**
- temporal surface
- orbital surface
- nasal bone
- zygomatic arch
- zygomatic bone
- infraorbital foramen
- inferior nasal concha
- nasal septum
- maxilla
- intermaxillary suture

- frontal bone
- coronal suture
- nasion
- lesser wing of sphenoid bone
- temporal bone
- superior orbital fissure
- optic canal
- nasolacrimal canal
- inferior orbital fissure
- zygomaticomaxillary suture
- vomer
- anterior nasal spine
- mandible
- mental foramen

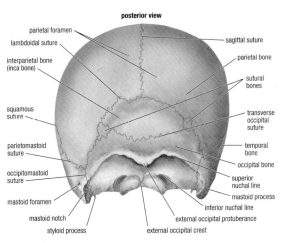

posterior view

- parietal foramen
- lambdoidal suture
- interparietal bone (inca bone)
- squamous suture
- parietomastoid suture
- occipitomastoid suture
- mastoid foramen
- mastoid notch
- styloid process

- sagittal suture
- parietal bone
- sutural bones
- transverse occipital suture
- temporal bone
- occipital bone
- superior nuchal line
- mastoid process
- inferior nuchal line
- external occipital protuberance
- external occipital crest

Cerebral hemispheres

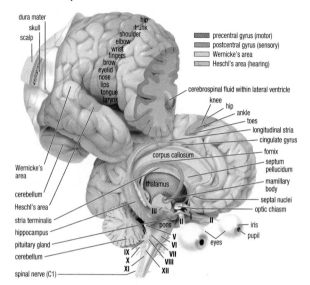

- dura mater
- skull
- scalp
- hip
- trunk
- shoulder
- elbow
- wrist
- fingers
- brow
- eyelid
- nose
- lips
- tongue
- larynx

- precentral gyrus (motor)
- postcentral gyrus (sensory)
- Wernicke's area
- Heschl's area (hearing)

- cerebrospinal fluid within lateral ventricle
- knee
- hip
- ankle
- toes
- longitudinal stria
- cingulate gyrus
- fornix
- septum pellucidum
- mamillary body
- septal nuclei
- optic chiasm
- iris
- pupil
- eyes

- corpus callosum
- thalamus
- Wernicke's area
- cerebellum
- Heschl's area
- stria terminalis
- hippocampus
- pituitary gland
- cerebellum
- spinal nerve (C1)
- III
- II
- II
- V
- VI
- VII
- VIII
- XII
- IX
- X
- XI
- pons

key

cranial nerves

I olfactory nerve — smell	**VII** facial nerve — face (motor), taste
II optic nerve — sight	**VIII** vestibulocochlear nerve — hearing and balance
III oculomotor — eye movement	**IX** glossopharyngeal nerve — swallowing, taste, sensation
IV trochlear nerve — eye movement (not illustrated)	**X** vagus nerve — gastrointestinal tract, swallowing, heart rate, peristalsis
V trigeminal nerve — face (sensory)	**XI** accessory nerve — shoulder muscles
VI abducens nerve — eye movement	**XII** hypoglossal nerve — tongue

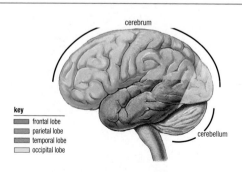

- cerebrum
- cerebellum

key

- frontal lobe
- parietal lobe
- temporal lobe
- occipital lobe

Anatomy of heart

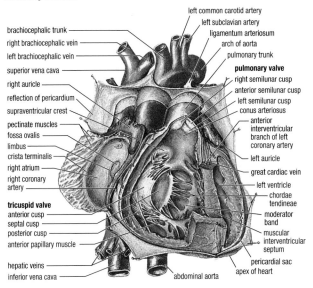

brachiocephalic trunk

right brachiocephalic vein

left brachiocephalic vein

superior vena cava

right auricle

reflection of pericardium

supraventricular crest

pectinate muscles

fossa ovalis

limbus

crista terminalis

right atrium

right coronary artery

tricuspid valve

anterior cusp

septal cusp

posterior cusp

anterior papillary muscle

hepatic veins

inferior vena cava

left common carotid artery

left subclavian artery

ligamentum arteriosum

arch of aorta

pulmonary trunk

pulmonary valve

right semilunar cusp

anterior semilunar cusp

left semilunar cusp

conus arteriosus

anterior interventricular branch of left coronary artery

left auricle

great cardiac vein

left ventricle

chordae tendineae

moderator band

muscular interventricular septum

pericardial sac

apex of heart

abdominal aorta

Male and female urogenital systems

sagittal section

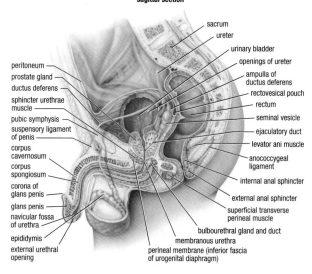

- sacrum
- ureter
- urinary bladder
- openings of ureter
- ampulla of ductus deferens
- rectovesical pouch
- rectum
- seminal vesicle
- ejaculatory duct
- levator ani muscle
- anococcygeal ligament
- internal anal sphincter
- external anal sphincter
- superficial transverse perineal muscle
- bulbourethral gland and duct
- membranous urethra
- perineal membrane (inferior fascia of urogenital diaphragm)

- peritoneum
- prostate gland
- ductus deferens
- sphincter urethrae muscle
- pubic symphysis
- suspensory ligament of penis
- corpus cavernosum
- corpus spongiosum
- corona of glans penis
- glans penis
- navicular fossa of urethra
- epididymis
- external urethral opening

medial section

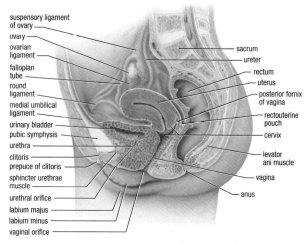

- suspensory ligament of ovary
- ovary
- ovarian ligament
- fallopian tube
- round ligament
- medial umbilical ligament
- urinary bladder
- pubic symphysis
- urethra
- clitoris
- prepuce of clitoris
- sphincter urethrae muscle
- urethral orifice
- labium majus
- labium minus
- vaginal orifice

- sacrum
- ureter
- rectum
- uterus
- posterior fornix of vagina
- rectouterine pouch
- cervix
- levator ani muscle
- vagina
- anus

Skeletal anatomy, anterior view

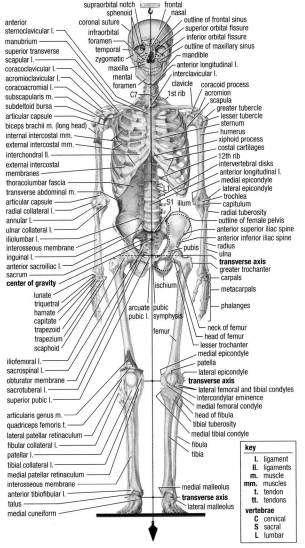

supraorbital notch
sphenoid
frontal
nasal
anterior
sternoclavicular l.
manubrium
superior transverse
scapular l.
coracoclavicular l.
acromioclavicular l.
coracoacromial l.
subscapularis m.
subdeltoid bursa
articular capsule
biceps brachii m. (long head)
internal intercostal mm.
external intercostal mm.
interchondral ll.
external intercostal
membranes
thoracolumbar fascia
transverse abdominal m.
articular capsule
radial collateral l.
annular l.
ulnar collateral l.
iliolumbar l.
interosseous membrane
inguinal l.
anterior sacroiliac l.
sacrum
center of gravity

coronal suture
infraorbital
foramen
temporal
zygomatic
maxilla
mental
foramen
C7

outline of frontal sinus
superior orbital fissure
inferior orbital fissure
outline of maxillary sinus
mandible
anterior longitudinal l.
interclavicular l.
clavicle   coracoid process
1st rib   acromion
scapula
greater tubercle
lesser tubercle
sternum
humerus
xiphoid process
costal cartilages
12th rib
intervertebral disks
anterior longitudinal l.
medial epicondyle
lateral epicondyle
trochlea
capitulum
radial tuberosity
outline of female pelvis
anterior superior iliac spine
anterior inferior iliac spine
radius
ulna
transverse axis
greater trochanter
carpals
metacarpals

L1
S1 ilium

pubis

lunate
triquetral
hamate
capitate
trapezoid
trapezium
scaphoid

iliofemoral l.
sacrospinal l.
obturator membrane
sacrotuberal l.
superior pubic l.

articularis genus m.
quadriceps femoris t.
lateral patellar retinaculum
fibular collateral l.
patellar l.
tibial collateral l.
medial patellar retinaculum
interosseous membrane
anterior tibiofibular l.
talus
medial cuneiform

arcuate
pubic l.
femur

pubic
symphysis

phalanges

neck of femur
head of femur
lesser trochanter
medial epicondyle
patella
lateral epicondyle
transverse axis
lateral femoral and tibial condyles
intercondylar eminence
medial femoral condyle
head of fibula
tibial tuberosity
medial tibial condyle
fibula
tibia

medial malleolus
transverse axis
lateral malleolus

ischium

key

l.	ligament
ll.	ligaments
m.	muscle
mm.	muscles
t.	tendon
tt.	tendons
vertebrae	
C	cervical
S	sacral
L	lumbar

Skeletal anatomy, posterior view

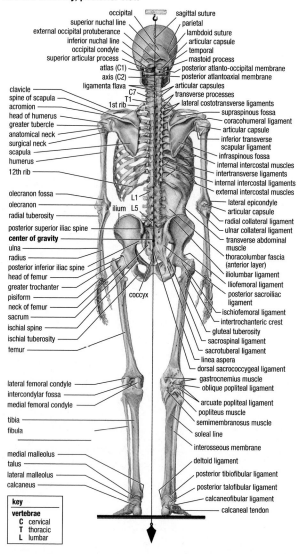

occipital
superior nuchal line
external occipital protuberance
inferior nuchal line
occipital condyle
superior articular process
atlas (C1)
axis (C2)
ligamenta flava
C7
T1
1st rib

sagittal suture
parietal
lambdoid suture
articular capsule
temporal
mastoid process
posterior atlanto-occipital membrane
posterior atlantoaxial membrane
articular capsules
transverse processes
lateral costotransverse ligaments
suprasrinous fossa
coracohumeral ligament
articular capsule
inferior transverse
scapular ligament
infraspinous fossa
internal intercostal muscles
intertransverse ligaments
internal intercostal ligaments
external intercostal muscles

clavicle
spine of scapula
acromion
head of humerus
greater tubercle
anatomical neck
surgical neck
scapula
humerus
12th rib

olecranon fossa
olecranon
radial tuberosity
posterior superior iliac spine
center of gravity
ulna
radius
posterior inferior iliac spine
head of femur
greater trochanter
pisiform
neck of femur
sacrum
ischial spine
ischial tuberosity
femur

L1
ilium L5

coccyx

lateral epicondyle
articular capsule
radial collateral ligament
ulnar collateral ligament
transverse abdominal
muscle
thoracolumbar fascia
(anterior layer)
iliolumbar ligament
iliofemoral ligament
posterior sacroiliac
ligament
ischiofemoral ligament
intertrochanteric crest
gluteal tuberosity
sacrospinal ligament
sacrotuberal ligament
linea aspera
dorsal sacrococcygeal ligament

lateral femoral condyle
intercondylar fossa
medial femoral condyle

tibia
fibula

gastrocnemius muscle
oblique popliteal ligament
arcuate popliteal ligament
popliteus muscle
semimembranosus muscle
soleal line

interosseous membrane

medial malleolus
talus
lateral malleolus
calcaneus

deltoid ligament
posterior tibiofibular ligament
posterior talofibular ligament
calcaneofibular ligament
calcaneal tendon

key
vertebrae
C cervical
T thoracic
L lumbar

Muscular system, anterior view

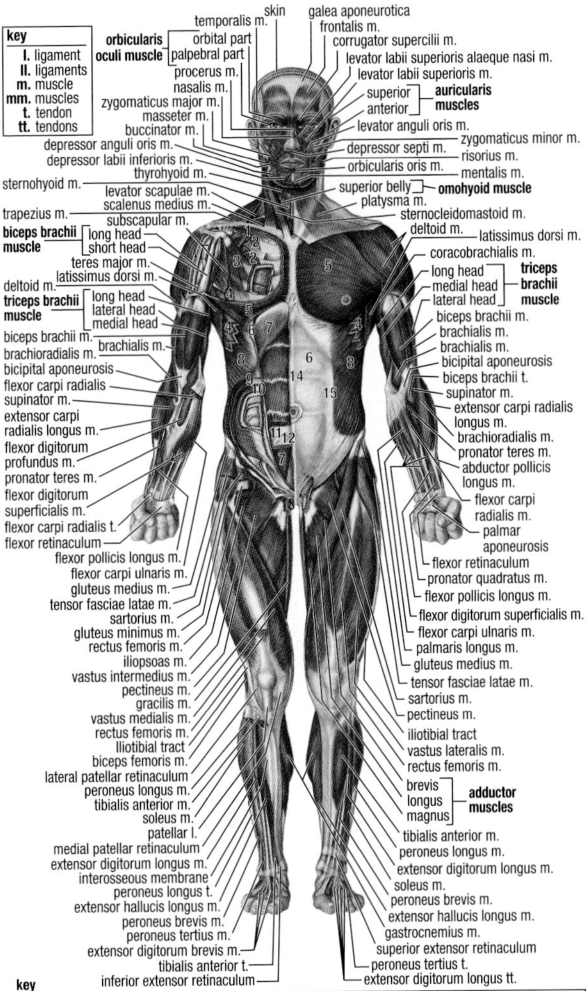
key
l. ligament
ll. ligaments
m. muscle
mm. muscles
t. tendon
tt. tendons
skin
temporalis m.
galea aponeurotica
frontalis m.
orbicularis oculi muscle
orbital part
palpebral part
corrugator supercilii m.
levator labii superioris alaeque nasi m.
levator labii superioris m.
procerus m.
nasalis m.
superior
anterior
auricularis muscles
zygomaticus major m.
masseter m.
buccinator m.
levator anguli oris m.
depressor anguli oris m.
zygomaticus minor m.
depressor septi m.
depressor labii inferioris m.
risorius m.
orbicularis oris m.
thyrohyoid m.
mentalis m.
sternohyoid m.
levator scapulae m.
superior belly
omohyoid muscle
scalenus medius m.
platysma m.
trapezius m.
sternocleidomastoid m.
subscapular m.
deltoid m.
latissimus dorsi m.
biceps brachii muscle
long head
short head
coracobrachialis m.
teres major m.
latissimus dorsi m.
long head
medial head
lateral head
triceps brachii muscle
deltoid m.
triceps brachii muscle
long head
lateral head
medial head
biceps brachii m.
brachialis m.
biceps brachii m.
brachialis m.
brachialis m.
brachioradialis m.
bicipital aponeurosis
bicipital aponeurosis
biceps brachii t.
flexor carpi radialis
supinator m.
supinator m.
extensor carpi radialis longus m.
extensor carpi radialis longus m.
brachioradialis m.
flexor digitorum profundus m.
pronator teres m.
pronator teres m.
abductor pollicis longus m.
flexor digitorum superficialis m.
flexor carpi radialis m.
flexor carpi radialis t.
palmar aponeurosis
flexor retinaculum
flexor retinaculum
flexor pollicis longus m.
pronator quadratus m.
flexor carpi ulnaris m.
flexor pollicis longus m.
gluteus medius m.
tensor fasciae latae m.
flexor digitorum superficialis m.
sartorius m.
flexor carpi ulnaris m.
gluteus minimus m.
palmaris longus m.
rectus femoris m.
gluteus medius m.
iliopsoas m.
vastus intermedius m.
tensor fasciae latae m.
pectineus m.
sartorius m.
gracilis m.
pectineus m.
vastus medialis m.
iliotibial tract
rectus femoris m.
vastus lateralis m.
Iliotibial tract
rectus femoris m.
biceps femoris m.
lateral patellar retinaculum
brevis
longus
magnus
adductor muscles
peroneus longus m.
tibialis anterior m.
soleus m.
tibialis anterior m.
patellar l.
peroneus longus m.
medial patellar retinaculum
extensor digitorum longus m.
extensor digitorum longus m.
interosseous membrane
soleus m.
peroneus longus t.
peroneus brevis m.
extensor hallucis longus m.
extensor hallucis longus m.
peroneus brevis m.
gastrocnemius m.
peroneus tertius m.
superior extensor retinaculum
extensor digitorum brevis m.
peroneus tertius t.
tibialis anterior t.
extensor digitorum longus tt.
inferior extensor retinaculum
1
2
2
3
4
5
5
4
6
7
4
8
6
8
9
10
14
15
11
12
7
13

key

- **1** subclavius m.
- **2** external intercostal mm.
- **3** pectoralis minor m.
- **4** serratus anterior m.
- **5** pectoralis major m.
- **6** rectus sheath (anterior layer)
- **7** rectus abdominis m.
- **8** external abdominal oblique m.
- **9** internal abdominal oblique m.
- **10** transversus abdominis m.
- **11** rectus sheath (posterior layer)
- **12** arcuate line
- **13** cremaster m.
- **14** linea alba
- **15** aponeurosis of external abdominal oblique m.

Muscular system, posterior view

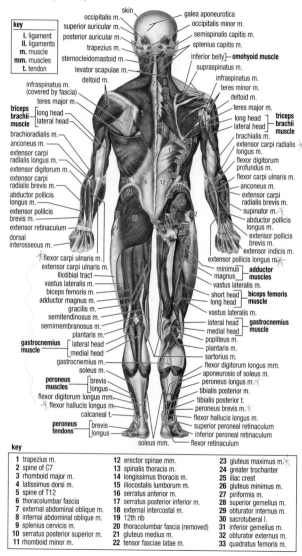

key
- **l.** ligament
- **ll.** ligaments
- **m.** muscle
- **mm.** muscles
- **t.** tendon

skin
galea aponeurotica
occipitalis m.
occipitalis minor m.
superior auricular m.
semispinalis capitis m.
posterior auricular m.
splenius capitis m.
trapezius m.
inferior belly]— **omohyoid muscle**
sternocleidomastoid m.
supraspinatus m.
levator scapulae m.
deltoid m.
infraspinatus m.
infraspinatus m. (covered by fascia)
teres minor m.
teres major m.
deltoid m.
teres major m.
triceps brachii muscle [long head, lateral head
long head] **triceps brachii muscle**
lateral head
brachioradialis m.
brachialis m.
anconeus m.
extensor carpi radialis longus m.
extensor carpi radialis longus m.
flexor digitorum profundus m.
extensor digitorum m.
flexor carpi ulnaris m.
extensor carpi radialis brevis m.
anconeus m.
abductor pollicis longus m.
extensor carpi radialis brevis m.
extensor pollicis brevis m.
supinator m.
extensor retinaculum
abductor pollicis longus m.
dorsal interosseous m.
extensor pollicis brevis m.
extensor indicis m.
flexor carpi ulnaris m.
extensor pollicis longus m.
extensor carpi ulnaris m.
minimus] **adductor muscles**
Iliotibial tract
magnus
vastus lateralis m.
vastus lateralis m.
biceps femoris m.
short head] **biceps femoris muscle**
adductor magnus m.
long head
gracilis m.
vastus lateralis m.
semitendinosus m.
lateral head] **gastrocnemius muscle**
semimembranosus m.
medial head
plantaris m.
popliteus m.
gastrocnemius muscle [lateral head, medial head
plantaris m.
gastrocnemius m.
sartorius m.
soleus m.
flexor digitorum longus mm.
aponeurosis of soleus m.
peroneus muscles [brevis, longus
peroneus longus m.
tibialis posterior m.
flexor digitorum longus mm.
tibialis posterior t.
flexor hallucis longus m.
peroneus brevis m.
calcaneal t.
flexor hallucis longus m.
peroneus tendons [brevis, longus
superior peroneal retinaculum
inferior peroneal retinaculum
soleus mm.
flexor retinaculum

key

1 trapezius m.	12 erector spinae mm.	23 gluteus maximus m.
2 spine of C7	13 spinalis thoracis m.	24 greater trochanter
3 rhomboid major m.	14 longissimus thoracis m.	25 iliac crest
4 latissimus dorsi m.	15 iliocostalis lumborum m.	26 gluteus minimus m.
5 spine of T12	16 serratus anterior m.	27 piriformis m.
6 thoracolumbar fascia	17 serratus posterior inferior m.	28 superior gemellus m.
7 external abdominal oblique m.	18 external intercostal m.	29 obturator internus m.
8 internal abdominal oblique m.	19 12th rib	30 sacrotuberal l.
9 splenius cervicis m.	20 thoracolumbar fascia (removed)	31 inferior gemellus m.
10 serratus posterior superior m.	21 gluteus medius m.	32 obturator externus m.
11 rhomboid minor m.	22 tensor fasciae latae m.	33 quadratus femoris m.

Spinal and cranial nerves

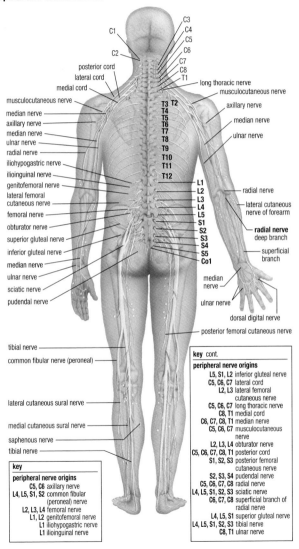

C1
C2
C3
C4
C5
C6
C7
C8
T1

posterior cord
lateral cord
medial cord
musculocutaneous nerve
median nerve
axillary nerve
median nerve
ulnar nerve
radial nerve
iliohypogastric nerve
ilioinguinal nerve
genitofemoral nerve
lateral femoral
cutaneous nerve
femoral nerve
obturator nerve
superior gluteal nerve
inferior gluteal nerve
median nerve
ulnar nerve
sciatic nerve
pudendal nerve

T2
T3
T4
T5
T6
T7
T8
T9
T10
T11
T12
L1
L2
L3
L4
L5
S1
S2
S3
S4
S5
Co1

long thoracic nerve
musculocutaneous nerve
axillary nerve
median nerve
ulnar nerve

radial nerve

lateral cutaneous
nerve of forearm

radial nerve
deep branch
superficial
branch

median
nerve

ulnar nerve

dorsal digital nerve
posterior femoral cutaneous nerve

tibial nerve
common fibular nerve (peroneal)

lateral cutaneous sural nerve

medial cutaneous sural nerve

saphenous nerve
tibial nerve

key
peripheral nerve origins
C5, C6 axillary nerve
L4, L5, S1, S2 common fibular
(peroneal) nerve
L2, L3, L4 femoral nerve
L1, L2 genitofemoral nerve
L1 iliohypogastric nerve
L1 ilioinguinal nerve

key cont.
peripheral nerve origins
L5, S1, L2 inferior gluteal nerve
C5, C6, C7 lateral cord
L2, L3 lateral femoral
cutaneous nerve
C5, C6, C7 long thoracic nerve
C8, T1 medial cord
C6, C7, C8, T1 median nerve
C5, C6, C7 musculocutaneous
nerve
L2, L3, L4 obturator nerve
C5, C6, C7, C8, T1 posterior cord
S1, S2, S3 posterior femoral
cutaneous nerve
S2, S3, S4 pudendal nerve
C5, C6, C7, C8 radial nerve
L4, L5, S1, S2, S3 sciatic nerve
C6, C7, C8 superficial branch of
radial nerve
L4, L5, S1 superior gluteal nerve
L4, L5, S1, S2, S3 tibial nerve
C8, T1 ulnar nerve

Arterial system, anterior view

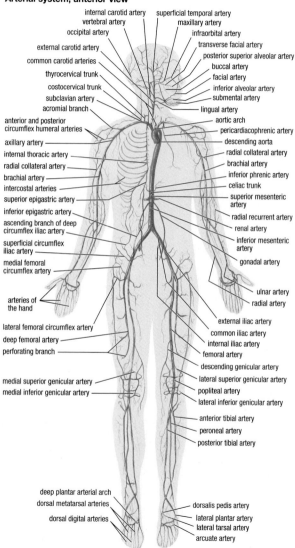

internal carotid artery
vertebral artery
occipital artery
external carotid artery
common carotid arteries
thyrocervical trunk
costocervical trunk
subclavian artery
acromial branch
anterior and posterior circumflex humeral arteries
axillary artery
internal thoracic artery
radial collateral artery
brachial artery
intercostal arteries
superior epigastric artery
inferior epigastric artery
ascending branch of deep circumflex iliac artery
superficial circumflex iliac artery
medial femoral circumflex artery
arteries of the hand
lateral femoral circumflex artery
deep femoral artery
perforating branch
medial superior genicular artery
medial inferior genicular artery
deep plantar arterial arch
dorsal metatarsal arteries
dorsal digital arteries

superficial temporal artery
maxillary artery
infraorbital artery
transverse facial artery
posterior superior alveolar artery
buccal artery
facial artery
inferior alveolar artery
submental artery
lingual artery
aortic arch
pericardiacophrenic artery
descending aorta
radial collateral artery
brachial artery
inferior phrenic artery
celiac trunk
superior mesenteric artery
radial recurrent artery
renal artery
inferior mesenteric artery
gonadal artery
ulnar artery
radial artery
external iliac artery
common iliac artery
internal iliac artery
femoral artery
descending genicular artery
lateral superior genicular artery
popliteal artery
lateral inferior genicular artery
anterior tibial artery
peroneal artery
posterior tibial artery
dorsalis pedis artery
lateral plantar artery
lateral tarsal artery
arcuate artery

Venous system, anterior view

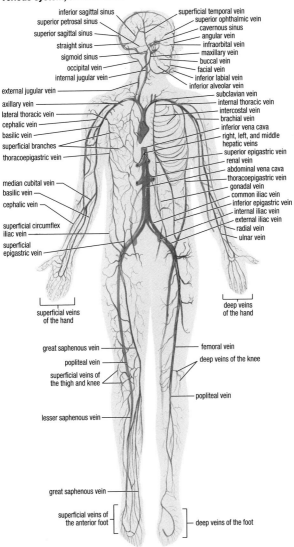

inferior sagittal sinus
superior petrosal sinus
superior sagittal sinus
straight sinus
sigmoid sinus
occipital vein
internal jugular vein
external jugular vein
axillary vein
lateral thoracic vein
cephalic vein
basilic vein
superficial branches
thoracoepigastric vein
median cubital vein
basilic vein
cephalic vein
superficial circumflex
iliac vein
superficial
epigastric vein

superficial temporal vein
superior ophthalmic vein
cavernous sinus
angular vein
infraorbital vein
maxillary vein
buccal vein
facial vein
inferior labial vein
inferior alveolar vein
subclavian vein
internal thoracic vein
intercostal vein
brachial vein
inferior vena cava
right, left, and middle
hepatic veins
superior epigastric vein
renal vein
abdominal vena cava
thoracoepigastric vein
gonadal vein
common iliac vein
inferior epigastric vein
internal iliac vein
external iliac vein
radial vein
ulnar vein

superficial veins
of the hand

deep veins
of the hand

great saphenous vein
popliteal vein
superficial veins of
the thigh and knee

lesser saphenous vein

great saphenous vein

superficial veins of
the anterior foot

femoral vein
deep veins of the knee

popliteal vein

deep veins of the foot

Lymphatic system, anterior view

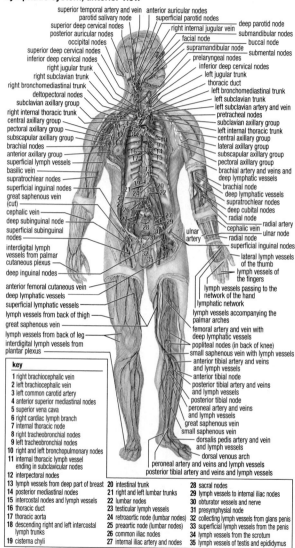

superior temporal artery and vein — anterior auricular nodes
parotid salivary node — superficial parotid nodes
superior deep cervical nodes — deep parotid node
posterior auricular nodes — right internal jugular vein — submandibular nodes
occipital nodes — facial node — buccal node
superior deep cervical nodes — supramandibular node — submental nodes
inferior deep cervical nodes — prelaryngeal nodes
right jugular trunk — inferior deep cervical nodes
right subclavian trunk — left jugular trunk
right bronchomediastinal trunk — thoracic duct
deltopectoral nodes — left bronchomediastinal trunk
subclavian axillary group — left subclavian trunk
right internal thoracic nodes — left subclavian artery and vein
central axillary group — pretracheal nodes
pectoral axillary group — subclavian axillary group
subscapular axillary group — left internal thoracic trunk
brachial nodes — central axillary group
anterior axillary group — lateral axillary group
superficial lymph vessels — subscapular axillary group
basilic vein — pectoral axillary group
supratrochlear nodes — brachial artery and veins and deep lymphatic vessels
superficial inguinal nodes — brachial node
great saphenous vein (cut) — deep lymphatic vessels
cephalic vein — supratrochlear nodes
deep subinguinal node — deep cubital nodes
superficial subinguinal nodes — radial node
interdigital lymph vessels from palmar cutaneous plexus — cephalic vein — radial artery
deep inguinal nodes — ulnar node
anterior femoral cutaneous vein — ulnar artery — radial artery
deep lymphatic vessels — superficial inguinal nodes
superficial lymphatic vessels — lateral lymph vessels of the thumb
lymph vessels from back of thigh — lymph vessels of the fingers
great saphenous vein — lymph vessels passing to the network of the hand
lymph vessels from back of leg — lymphatic network
interdigital lymph vessels from plantar plexus — lymph vessels accompanying the palmar arches
femoral artery and vein with deep lymphatic vessels
popliteal nodes (in back of knee)
small saphenous vein with lymph vessels
anterior tibial artery and veins and lymph vessels
anterior tibial node
posterior tibial artery and veins and lymph vessels
posterior tibial node
peroneal artery and veins and lymph vessels
great saphenous vein
small saphenous vein
dorsalis pedis artery and vein and lymph vessels
dorsal venous arch
peroneal artery and veins and lymph vessels
posterior tibial artery and veins and lymph vessels

key

1 right brachiocephalic vein
2 left brachiocephalic vein
3 left common carotid artery
4 anterior superior mediastinal nodes
5 superior vena cava
6 right cardiac lymph branch
7 internal thoracic node
8 right tracheobronchial nodes
9 left tracheobronchial nodes
10 right and left bronchopulmonary nodes
11 internal thoracic lymph vessel ending in subclavicular nodes
12 interpectoral nodes
13 lymph vessels from deep part of breast
14 posterior mediastinal nodes
15 intercostal nodes and lymph vessels
16 thoracic duct
17 thoracic aorta
18 descending right and left intercostal lymph trunks
19 cisterna chyli

20 intestinal trunk
21 right and left lumbar trunks
22 lumbar nodes
23 testicular lymph vessels
24 retroaortic node (lumbar nodes)
25 preaortic node (lumbar nodes)
26 common iliac nodes
27 internal iliac artery and nodes

28 sacral nodes
29 lymph vessels to internal iliac nodes
30 obturator vessels and nerve
31 presymphysial node
32 collecting lymph vessels from glans penis
33 superficial lymph vessels from the penis
34 lymph vessels from the scrotum
35 lymph vessels of testis and epididymus

Respiratory system, anterior view

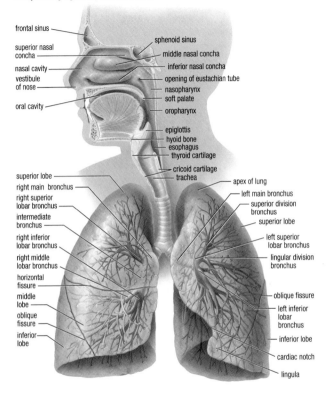

frontal sinus

sphenoid sinus

superior nasal concha

middle nasal concha

inferior nasal concha

nasal cavity

opening of eustachian tube

vestibule of nose

nasopharynx

soft palate

oral cavity

oropharynx

epiglottis

hyoid bone

esophagus

thyroid cartilage

cricoid cartilage

trachea

superior lobe

apex of lung

right main bronchus

left main bronchus

right superior lobar bronchus

superior division bronchus

intermediate bronchus

superior lobe

right inferior lobar bronchus

left superior lobar bronchus

right middle lobar bronchus

lingular division bronchus

horizontal fissure

middle lobe

oblique fissure

oblique fissure

left inferior lobar bronchus

inferior lobe

inferior lobe

cardiac notch

lingula

Upper digestive system, anterior view

nasal cavity

tongue
oropharynx

esophagus

liver

aorta

celiac trunk
stomach

gallbladder

portal vein

esophagus

diaphragm

stomach

Lower digestive system, anterior view

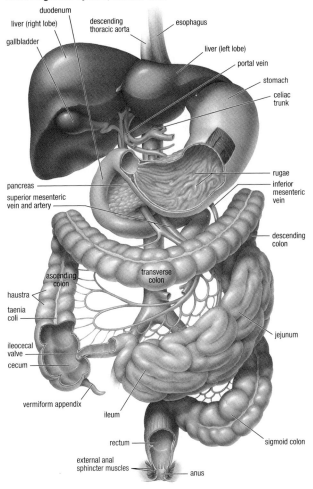

liver (right lobe)

duodenum

gallbladder

descending
thoracic aorta

esophagus

liver (left lobe)

portal vein

stomach

celiac
trunk

pancreas

superior mesenteric
vein and artery

rugae

inferior
mesenteric
vein

descending
colon

ascending
colon

transverse
colon

haustra

taenia
coli

jejunum

ileocecal
valve

cecum

vermiform appendix

ileum

rectum

sigmoid colon

external anal
sphincter muscles

anus

Urinary system, anterior view

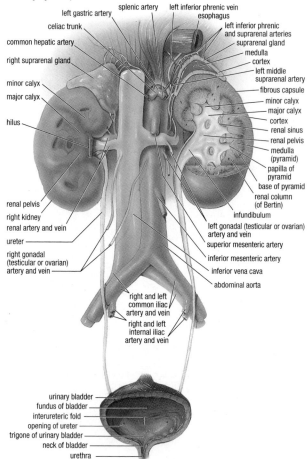

left gastric artery
splenic artery
left inferior phrenic vein
esophagus
celiac trunk
left inferior phrenic and suprarenal arteries
common hepatic artery
suprarenal gland
right suprarenal gland
medulla
cortex
left middle suprarenal artery
minor calyx
fibrous capsule
major calyx
minor calyx
major calyx
hilus
cortex
renal sinus
renal pelvis
medulla (pyramid)
papilla of pyramid
base of pyramid
renal column (of Bertin)
renal pelvis
infundibulum
right kidney
left gonadal (testicular or ovarian) artery and vein
renal artery and vein
superior mesenteric artery
ureter
inferior mesenteric artery
right gonadal (testicular or ovarian) artery and vein
inferior vena cava
abdominal aorta
right and left common iliac artery and vein
right and left internal iliac artery and vein
urinary bladder
fundus of bladder
interureteric fold
opening of ureter
trigone of urinary bladder
neck of bladder
urethra

CCS0908